# Eat Well, Weigh less

This is a Parragon book
This edition published in 2005

Parragon
Queen Street House
4 Queen Street
Bath, BA1 1HE, UK

Contributing Editor
Maggie Pannell

This edition designed by
Design Principals, Warminster



ISBN 1-40544-796-6
Printed in China

## DISCLAIMER

**The exercises and advice detailed in this book assume that you are a normally healthy adult. Therefore the author, publishers, their servants, or agents cannot accept responsibility for loss or damage suffered by individuals as a result of following advice or attempting an exercise or treatment referred to in this book. It is strongly recommended that individuals intending to undertake an exercise programme and any change of diet do so following consultation with their medical practitioner.**

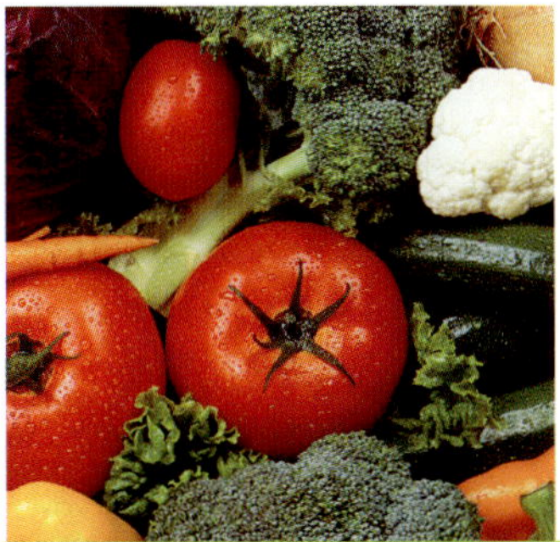

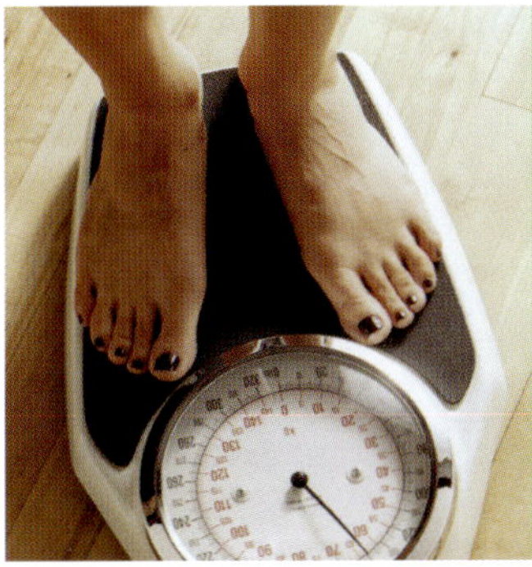

# Eat Well, Weigh less

a realistic and
practical healthy
eating plan that
makes dieting easy
and enjoyable

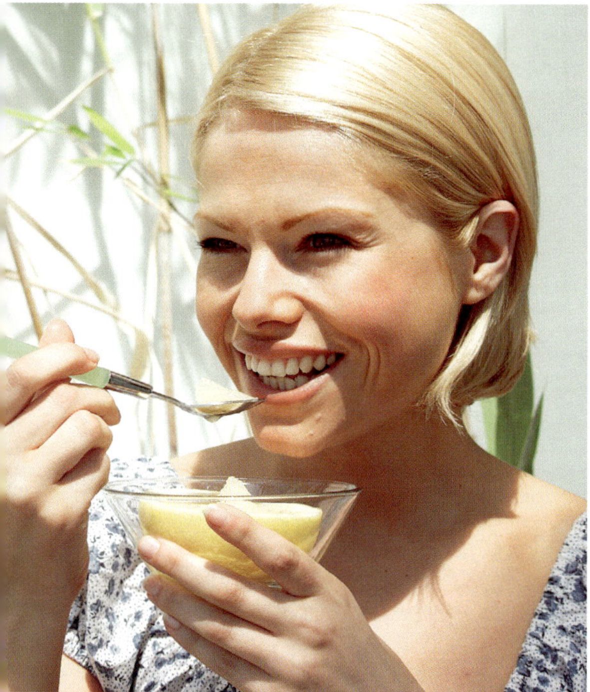

A diet including plenty of fruit and vegetables will be rich in vitamin C.

## Teeth

- A healthy diet is just as important as regular brushing and flossing when it comes to having clean, white, strong teeth.
- Healthy teeth require the same nutrients as strong bones, namely calcium, magnesium and vitamin D. Dairy products are the best source of calcium but other sources include nuts (especially almonds), seeds, fortified soya products (including tofu), canned sardines (with bones) and dark green leafy vegetables. Magnesium is found in wholegrain cereals, dried fruits, nuts, pulses and green vegetables.
- Looking after your gums is also essential. Foods rich in B group vitamins, beta-carotene vitamin C, zinc and folic acid will all help keep them healthy.
- Mouth ulcers are a sign that the immune system is compromised and that the body may be lacking in essential nutrients.
- Sugar is the biggest enemy of teeth, and it is the frequency that it is eaten that increases the likelihood of tooth decay.

## Nails

- Nails are made of a protein called keratin and should be strong, smooth and pink. Pale, brittle or ridged nails may be a sign of iron or zinc deficiency. If you suspect you are anaemic, ask your doctor for a blood test and boost your intake of iron-rich foods.
- Iron is found in offal, red meat, mussels, dried apricots, green leafy vegetables, pulses and fortified breakfast cereals.
- Eat plenty of vitamin C- rich foods at the same time to help absorb the iron.
- White spots on the nails may be a sign of zinc deficiency. Shellfish, seeds, lean meat, peanuts and wholegrain cereals are rich in zinc.

**A healthy outer self is an excellent indication of inner health and knowing that you look great is a wonderful confidence booster. Eating a well-balanced diet will not only help you get in shape but will also improve the condition of your skin, hair, teeth and nails.**

# Contents



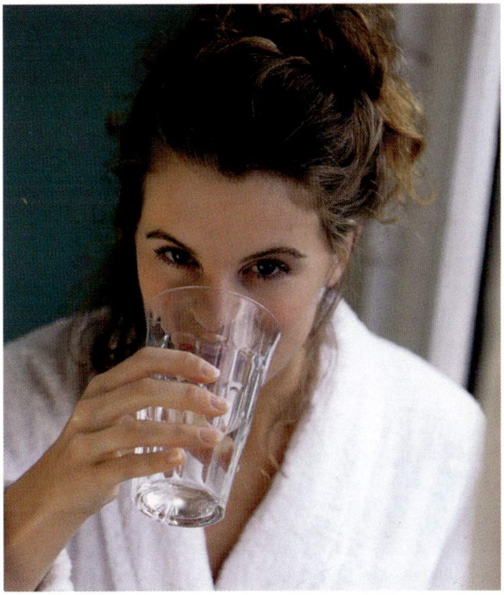

## Skin

- A good diet is the best action you can take to promote a glowing, healthy, blemish-free complexion. Choosing the right foods, rich in vitamins and essential fatty acids, will improve and revitalise the skin.
- The single most important 'nutrient' for a glowing complexion is water. Aim to drink 6-8 glasses a day to hydrate the skin and help flush out toxins. Stress, environmental pollution, sun and lack of sleep all take their toll on our skin and, of course, genetic make-up plays a part. Poor digestion, food intolerances and allergies can also cause or exacerbate skin disorders, such as acne and eczema.
- The skin is one of the major organs responsible for eliminating waste. A diet high in junk foods, laced with alcohol and cigarettes, means that it has to work harder to get rid of toxic waste products and can be overloaded with harmful toxins.

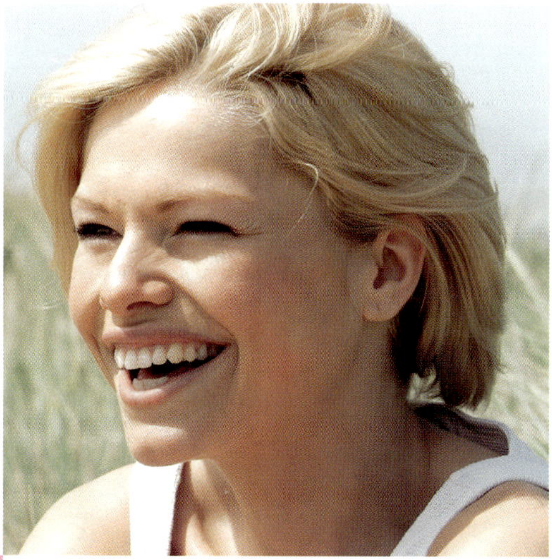

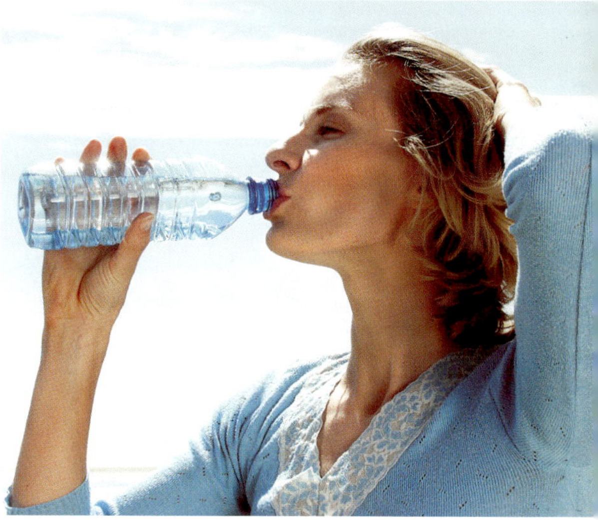

## Hair

- Dull, lack-lustre hair may be an indication that you are lacking in nutrients.
- Illness, stress or an emotional problem can all have a detrimental effect on your hair condition, which even a good haircut and the latest styling products won't be able to remedy.
- Over-exposure to hair-dyes and perming lotions sometimes causes hair and scalp problems, but a healthy, balanced diet will help to rectify the damage and boost condition.
- Essential fatty acids, found in oily fish, vegetable oils, nuts and seeds, can help prevent a dry, flaky scalp.
- Lean red meat, eggs, pulses, dried apricots and dark green leafy vegetables and fortified breakfast cereals are a good source of iron, which help counter hair loss.
- Drinking plenty of water can also improve the condition of your hair.

# How to do it sensibly

A sensible diet for weight loss is very similar to any healthy diet, except that fewer calories are consumed. Eating smaller portions and eating less fat will help reduce calories. There is no need, however, to count the calories in every mouthful.

Weight loss should be gradual. Losing more than about two lb (900g) per week is not effective in the long run. Quick, dramatic weight loss is usually the result of either losing water weight or of following a diet that is dangerously low in calories. Diets that have fewer than 1200 calories per day make your body go into starvation mode, reducing metabolism to conserve weight so that it is actually harder to lose weight. Very restrictive diets are also hard to stick to because they are dull.

Although most people will lose weight on a diet, few dieters manage to keep the weight off. Most people actually gain back the weight once they stop dieting, and even add a few extra pounds. The key to lasting weight loss is changing your eating habits, not just for the duration of the diet, but for the rest of your life. You need to teach yourself new, healthy eating habits and make them part of your life.

In order to teach yourself new habits, you need to educate yourself about foods. In general, fruits and vegetables, when cooked and served without added fat or sugar, can be eaten in large quantities. Changing to low-fat, dairy products is another good habit to start. Some cooking methods, such as deep-fat frying, sautéing and shallow frying, add fat to foods, while others such as baking, grilling, steaming, boiling and stir-frying in small amounts of oil, add very little. To add flavour, use citrus juices, herbs and spices, not butter, oil and salt.

For support and enthusiasm, encourage the whole family or a friend to follow the healthy eating plan with you. Joining a slimming club can also be helpful for moral support and encouragement but be sure to choose one that also advises a healthy weight loss programme. Methods that focus on gradual weight loss, healthy eating habits and realistic targets are healthier and work better in the long run.

When it comes to losing weight, fad diets don't work. You might have success on a diet for the period of time that you're on it, but more often than not, the weight comes back on afterwards. The solution is to follow a sensible, healthy eating plan that can be maintained for a lifetime. Height and weight charts will tell you if you are the right weight for your height, although your clothes not fitting and a frank look at yourself in a full-length mirror, will give you an honest assessment. Remember however, that muscle weighs more than fat so if you are muscular, your weight may be at the high end for your height.

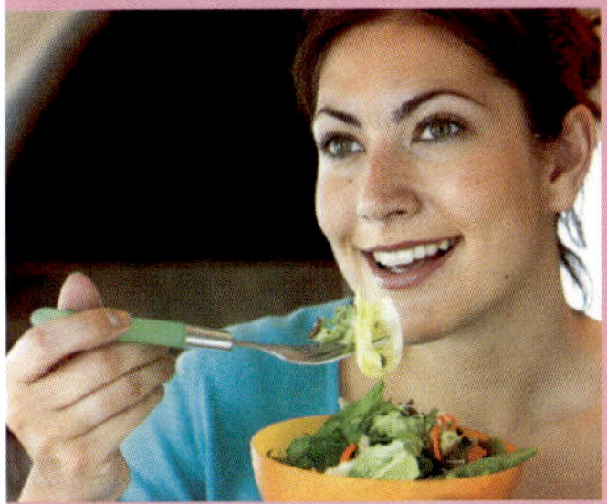

**Choosing a healthy diet is the best and most effective way to lose weight.**

## A summertime tan

There is no doubt that a slightly bronzed body looks healthier than a pale one and it gives the illusion of a slimmer outline too. But the health dangers related to over-exposure to the sun are well documented, so why not fake a tan? There are lots of good, easy-to-apply lotions and what's more you don't have to spend hours lying in the sun or worry about strap marks or peeling. Nor does it matter if the weather is poor, because come rain or shine, you can ensure your skin will have a healthy glow.

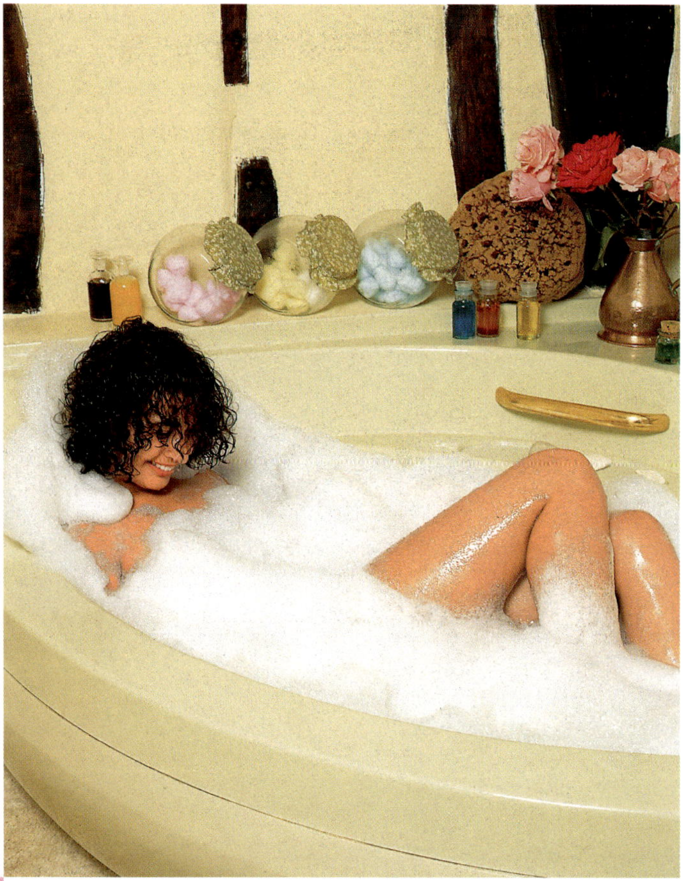

## Retail therapy

There's nothing like a little fashion shopping to perk up your spirits. So if you feel in need of some pampering or if you have had a particularly bad day, why not go out and treat yourself to something gorgeous. It doesn't have to be an expensive outfit. Anything from a new pair of earrings to some pretty lingerie can do wonders for lifting your mood.

## Pamper yourself

Set aside some time each day for a bit of personal TLC. It might be a relaxing soak with a luxurious bubble bath, a pedicure or manicure followed by a massage with a rich, creamy moisturiser or a fragrant face mask that really opens and cleans the pores and leaves your skin feeling fresh and radiant.

## Have some fun

As children, having fun came naturally but as adults we tend to forget how to have fun, and the more stressful and complex life becomes, the greater the need for the release that play provides. Having fun helps recharge your batteries so we can return to being an adult refreshed and ready for anything.

## REASONS WHY DIETS DON'T WORK

Here are some common reasons why diets fail. Follow the healthy eating guidelines and take regular exercise and you won't fall into these traps.

- Skipping breakfast – then filling up mid-morning on snack foods that tend to be high in fat and / or sugar.
- Making impulsive food choices.
- Not finding meals are adequately sustaining.
- Restricted food choices so the diet becomes dull and doesn't fit well with friends and family.
- Incompatibility with lifestyle.
- Eating between meals when bored, stressed or fed up.
- A sedentary lifestyle.
- Exercising on an empty stomach.
- Unrealistic goals.
- Lack of motivation.

## No more crash diets

Crash diets are very unsatisfactory – they usually make you feel miserable while you are doing them, and the effects are very short-lived. By changing your eating habits, you will no longer need to diet to lose weight. Instead you will be able to enjoy eating a variety of foods because you will know which foods to choose.

Exercising at the same time will help you lose weight faster, as well as toning your muscles. Since exercising burns up calories, and losing weight is the process of taking in fewer calories than you burn, burning extra calories through exercise makes sense.

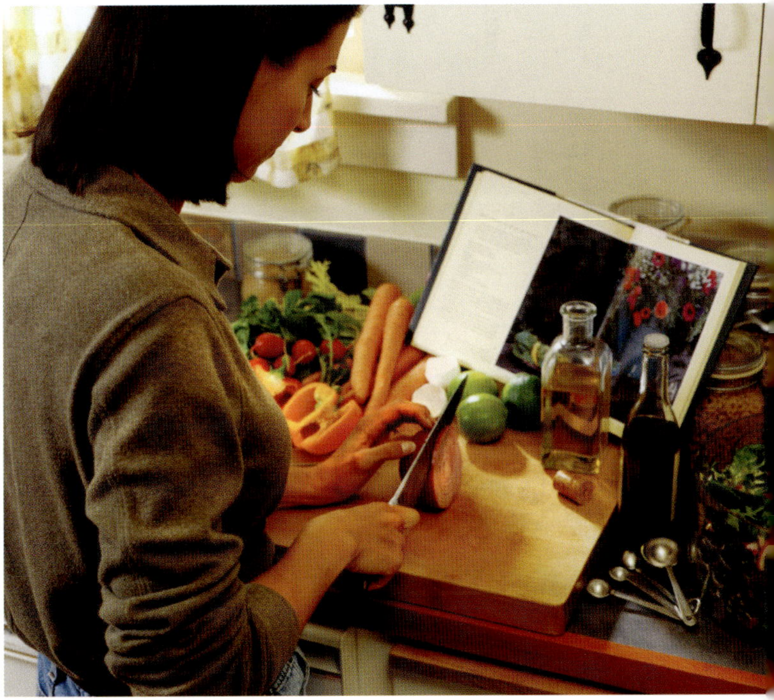

It may take a little longer to prepare fresh foods, but the health benefits make it a very worthwhile exercise.

# How to stay motivated

No matter how good your intentions at the beginning, there are bound to be days when you think, "Why bother? What is the point of it all?" We all have days like this and the way to cope with them is to recognise that hidden beneath those dull feelings are positive emotions lying in wait. So work hard to bring them to the fore by being pro-active in planning activities that will quickly snap you out of those negative thoughts and put you back on the straight and narrow.

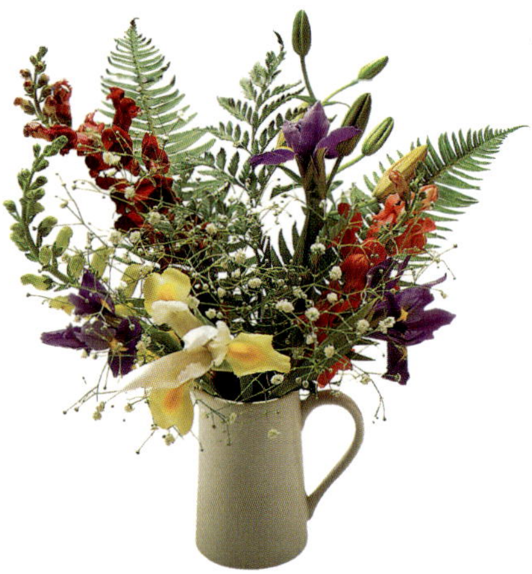

## Make a list

Write down a list of your own reasons for wanting to lose weight and shape up. Place it somewhere prominent like on the fridge door so that those aims and thoughts stay clearly focused in your mind.

## Gather support

It's never easy taking on a task alone so get your family and friends on to the healthy eating bandwagon too. They don't need to be dieting to lose weight but simply making changes to follow a healthier lifestyle.

## Get sponsored

Why not combine weight loss with a donation to your favourite charity? Get together a list of sponsors, decide on an amount per 1lb or 1 kg lost and ask a witness to weigh you at the start and finish. Just think what a high you'll get knowing what a good cause your efforts are going towards.

## Plan for a special occasion

Make sure that you always have something to look forward to. Leaf through your diary and find an upcoming event for which you'd like to look your best. It might be a wedding, christening or birthday, or a holiday you've booked. No matter what the occasion, it will give you something positive to aim for.

## Flower Power

Studies have shown that if you surround yourself with flowers, they can trigger off feelings of happiness, soothe away anxieties and improve your quality of life. So if your partner has not bought you a bunch recently, take the initiative and choose a pretty, scented bouquet for yourself.

# Weight & measurement checks

## Body mass index

The best way to work out your ideal body weight is to work out your body mass index (BMI). This is used to assess your body weight in relation to your height. It is closely related to your body fat percentage. Calculate your BMI using the simple formula below, then check the range in the guide to see whether you are underweight, the normal weight for your height, or overweight.

### CALCULATE YOUR BMI

Working in metric, divide your weight in kilograms by the square of your height

$$\text{BMI} = \frac{\text{Weight (kg)}}{\text{Height (m)}^2}$$

For example,
Weight = 65kg
Height = 1.65 x 1.65m = 2.72m,
BMI = 24 (65 ÷ 2.72)

**BMI under 19** Underweight. No need to lose weight, and you may need to gain a little weight if your BMI is significantly below 19. Consult your doctor if you are in doubt.

**BMI 19–25** Normal. Aim to keep your weight at this level. You're within healthy guidelines and the risk of weight-related health problems is minimal.

**BMI 25–29** Overweight. You are in the 'caution zone'. Your weight should not increase, and it's advisable to lose weight. There is a slightly increased risk of health problems.

**BMI 30–40** Officially obese. Reducing weight is highly recommended. The risk of weight-related health problems is increased.

**BMI over 40** Very important to lose weight. There is a high risk of weight-related health problems, and early death.

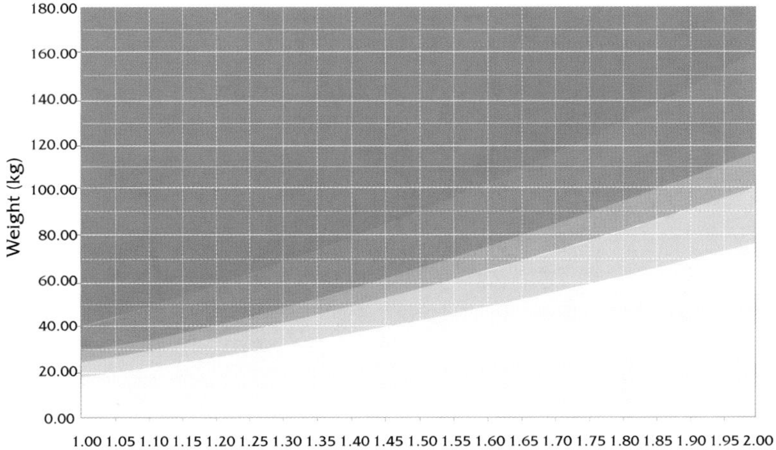


This body mass index chart gives you an indication of whether you are at risk of health problems.

# Exercises for reluctant keep-fitters

If you have been working all day, then possibly the last thing on your mind is doing anything more physical other than drinking a cup of tea. But it is still quite possible to tone and trim muscles even when sitting on the sofa.

**DID YOU KNOW?**
**Every 450g (1lb) of muscle in your body burns off 35 calories a day.**

## Head

Look directly in front and extend the back of the neck up and towards the ceiling whilst easing the shoulders down, keeping your jaw parallel with the floor. Hold for 5 seconds and repeat the other side.

## Shoulders

Ease both shoulders forwards and upwards, then back and down. The secret is to move through each new direction in one continuous circle, say it out loud: forward, upwards, backwards, downwards, making the circle as large as you are able.

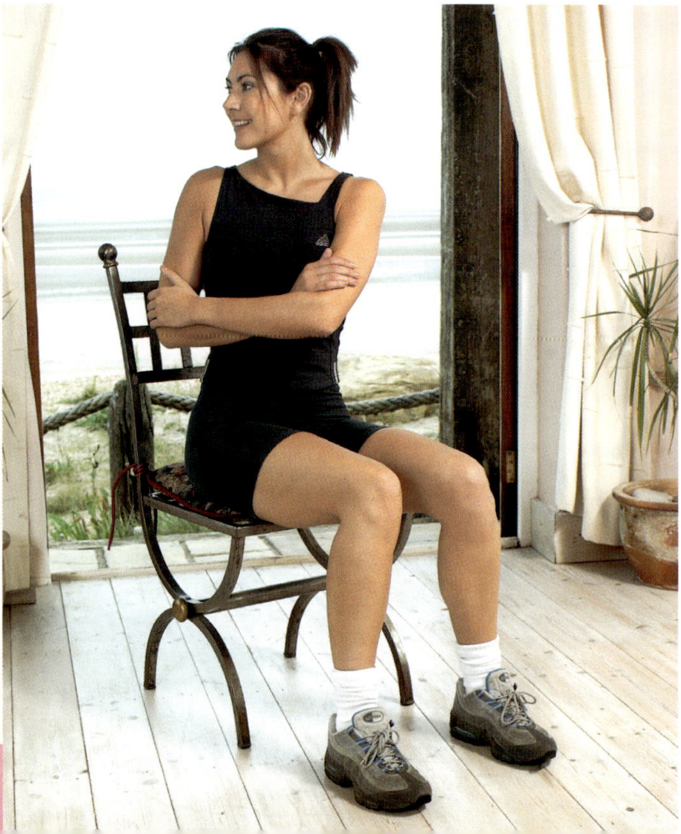

## Waist

1. Sit upright on a chair or stool with your legs and feet hip-width apart, and your knees directly over your ankles.
2. Put your arms at chest level, bent at the elbows with forearms resting on one another.
3. Twisting from the middle, slowly turn your head, shoulders and arms around to the left as far as possible, keeping your shoulders down throughout this move.
4. Return to the starting position and repeat the other side.

Repeat these exercises as often as possible. You can do them sitting at a desk or even in front of the T.V.

**TAKE CARE**
**If you have any chronic medical conditions or back problems, you should consult your doctor before starting any exercise programme.**

# Weight & measurement checks

## Measure your waist

Another way to check whether you are at any health risk because of your weight, is by measuring your waist circumference. Place the tape measure loosely around your waist, just above your tummy button.

- Waist circumference below 80cm (31½in) is classified as healthy.
- Waist circumference over 80cm (31½in) indicates a slight health risk.
- Waist circumference over 88cm (34½in) indicates a major health risk.

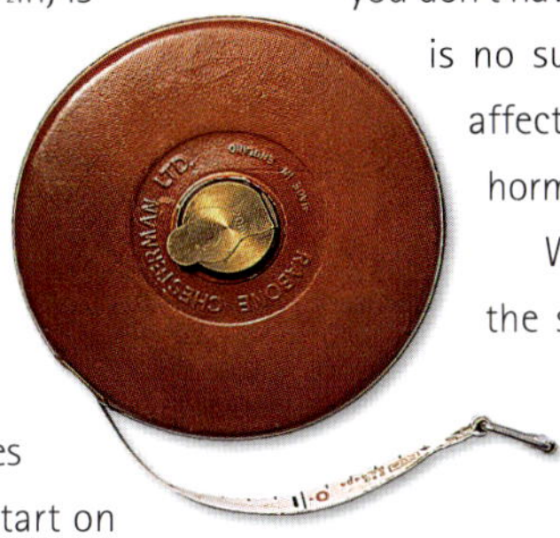

Using a tape measure is also a good way to monitor your efforts to lose inches from your bum and tum. Before you start on the programme, take one measurement across the level of your tummy button, and another around your hips, at the maximum protrusion of your bottom. Check the measurements at six- to eight-week intervals.

### FAT

**We all need a certain amount of fat to survive. It gives us shape, warmth and insulation, protects our internal organs and provides us with a reserve fuel supply. The problems arise when we store too much fat in the body from overeating and underactivity. The only way to lose it is through burning calories and eating sensibly. The fat cells don't disappear completely, but the amount of fat stored can increase/decrease depending on how well we eat and how much exercise we take.**

## Cellulite

Most women are familiar with what cellulite is – recent research revealed that more than 95 per cent of women over the age of 35 have it! It's that dimpled 'orange peel' skin that appears on women's thighs and buttocks. And you don't have to be overweight to get it – being thin is no sure-fire defence. Men are only rarely affected, because the structure of cellulite is hormonally controlled.

Women naturally need more fat around the stomach, hips, thighs and buttocks – without this, they wouldn't be able to sustain a pregnancy. Around every fat cell is a collagen support structure that keeps it together. In men, this particular structure is stronger because of the male sex hormone, testosterone. In women, the support structure is weaker and the cells pucker, producing an unsightly, dimpled effect – cellulite!

An inactive lifestyle contributes to the formation of fat and in women this often appears as cellulite in the legs. Diet is one of the most important factors in treating cellulite. Regular exercise is another – walking briskly, jogging/running, cycling and step or aerobic classes are ideal, as these burn lots of energy, the legs are toned and all the muscles are tightened. While swimming is an excellent form of exercise for burning fat, it's not so good for dealing with cellulite, as the body weight is supported while you're working out in the water. As with any aerobic exercise, to get the best result you need to work out for 20–30 minutes, three to five times a week.

## Swimming

Swimming works most of the major muscle groups and is an excellent aerobic exercise. It is the ideal exercise if you are overweight as the water supports the weight of your body. So even if you are very overweight, you'll find it easy to swim. It's good for people of all ages and all levels of fitness and is especially beneficial if you suffer from back pain or joint problems and therefore find other forms of exercise difficult. Either pop along to your nearest pool at any time to suit yourself or if you prefer a group session, check if there are any classes you'd like to attend. Most pools offer 'early bird' swims for early risers to swim before work, ladies only sessions, parent and baby classes and crèche facilities. To get the greatest benefit from swimming, you need to swim laps, using any stroke you choose, and build up your stamina by swimming up and down for as long as you can, without stopping.

## Yoga

It may sound rather odd thinking that yoga can help deal with cellulite, but those who practise yoga fervently very rarely suffer with it. It seems that all the stretching and flexing of muscles activates the circulation of blood and other fluids around the body.

It may be a good idea to see if there are any local yoga classes to join or why not visit the library to borrow some yoga books and a video to do at home.

### EXERCISING FOR NEW MUMS

After giving birth, most women find that their figure has lost some of its firmness and that the stomach, in particular remains rather flabby. Don't worry – with some gentle and regular exercising, those over-stretched abdominal muscles will soon return to normal and you'll be able to wear those figure-hugging clothes again. Don't set yourself an exhausting schedule, but ease yourself into a routine gently. Your health visitor will recommend specific postnatal exercises but simply taking the baby out for walks in the pram / buggy is good exercise. Yoga exercises are very good too.

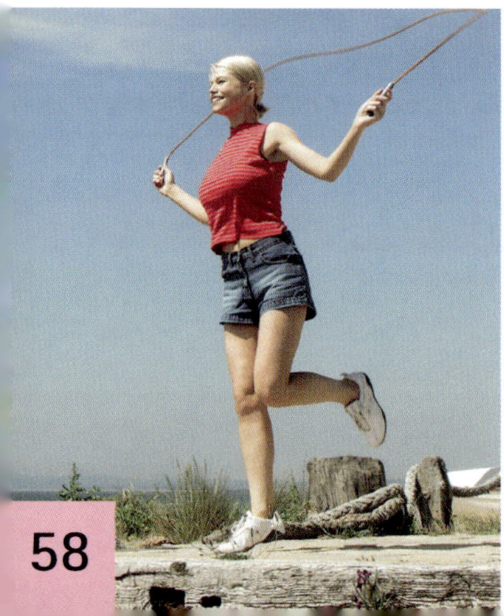

## Skipping

Indoors or outdoors, skipping is the ideal, all-over workout and perfect for stretching the leg muscles. It also works the heart, lungs and upper body to get a really good workout. You may have to start in bursts of 2-3 minutes, but you will be pleasantly surprised how quickly the body adapts to easily managing longer sessions. The beauty of skipping is that you can do it virtually anywhere at any time. All you need is a skipping rope that you can buy cheaply from any toy shop or department store, then off you go.

# Eating for the figure you want

**How would you like to get in shape with a diet that's easy and delicious to follow, fits in effortlessly with family, friends and a busy lifestyle and doesn't leave you feeling hungry? There is no magic formula. It's simply a matter of choosing a healthy diet.**

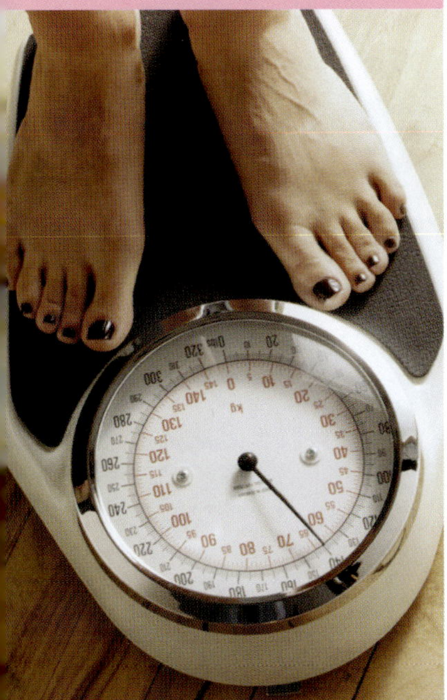

**Your weight on the scales may not be the best indication of how fit you are – muscle weighs more than fat.**

Balance and variety are the key to planning a healthy, figure-trimming diet. This means eating a good range of starchy carbohydrates, plenty of fruit and vegetables, moderate amounts of protein foods (meat, fish and alternatives) and moderate amounts of milk and dairy foods, to ensure you get the nutrients vital for good health. Foods that are high in fat and/or sugar should be limited as they are high in calories without providing much in the way of nutrient value and, if eaten too freely, pile on weight as well as causing various health problems. This is the group of foods that you need to restrict and regard as 'special treats', especially when dieting.

It's impossible to give exact amounts that you should eat, as everyone's requirements are different, depending on their gender, size, age and level of activity. However, the ideal proportions of foods from the five groups remain the same: -

- Fruit and vegetables – $^1/_3$ of daily intake
- Starchy carbohydrates – $^1/_3$ of daily intake
- Protein foods (meat, fish and alternatives) – $^1/_8$ of daily intake
- Milk & dairy foods – $^1/_6$ of daily intake
- Foods high in fat and /or sugar – strictly as occasional treats (see What to avoid on pgs 13 –15)

## Getting the balance right

All food provides energy, measured in calories (kcals) or joules (kJ). On average, women need around 2,000 calories a day while men need roughly 2,500 calories a day, depending on age, sex, body weight and lifestyle.

If you balance the amount of energy you take in with the amount of energy you use, your body weight will remain the same.

However, if you regularly take in more calories than you need, your body will convert the surplus to fat and you will steadily gain weight.

Conversely, to lose weight, you need to either eat fewer calories or take more exercise so your body will start to burn up its fat reserves. A combination of making healthy food choices together with becoming more active is the most effective method of dieting.

## Gardening

If you don't feel like doing anything beyond your home patch and you have a garden, then look no further for your daily exercise. Mow the lawn – it's great for toning up the abdominal muscles; how about pruning those high branches – no better exercise for toning the arms and back; or pull up weeds – it is the ideal answer for working on those thighs as you bend and straighten. It also helps to tone up buttocks and arms, and the bonus is that your garden looks good too.

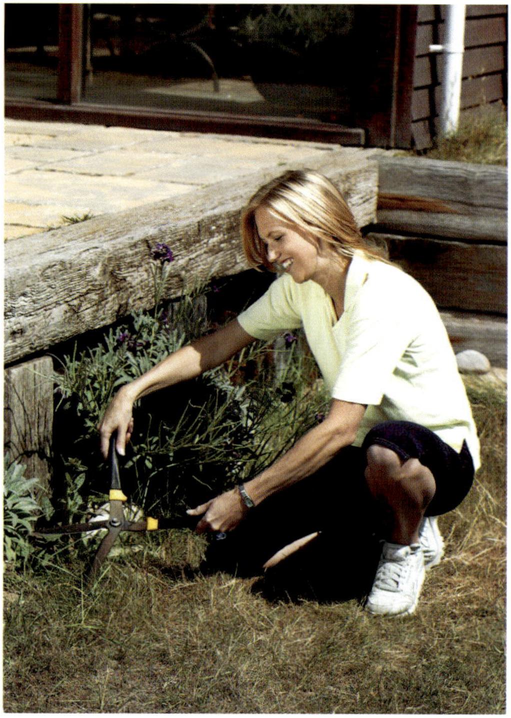

## Dancing

Whether you like ballroom dancing, salsa, ceroc (modern jive) or disco dancing, this hardly feels like exercise. But it is an excellent form of aerobic exercise and just goes to prove how much fun exercise can be. It's also something you can do socially with a partner or group of friends or why not sign up for classes and go along to meet new people.

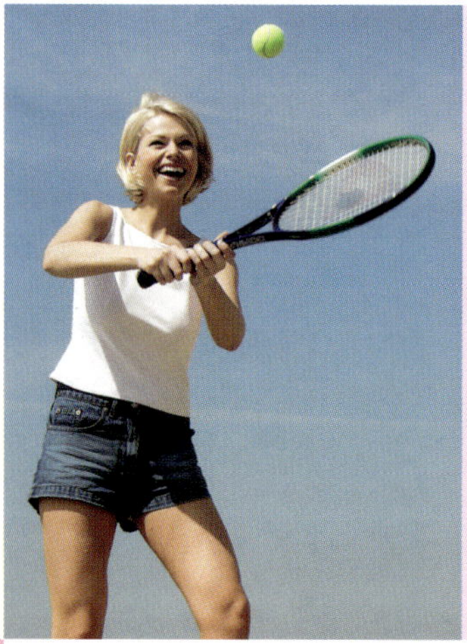

## Badminton / tennis / squash

Find out about clubs and sports facilities at your local library or search the internet for what's happening in your area. Many upper schools and colleges run a varied programme of adult education classes, including a wide range of sports. Badminton, tennis and squash are very popular sports for both men and women and classes are a fun way of meeting new people. If you're a beginner, start playing at your own level with others of a similar standard. Then as your game improves, the exercise will become more aerobic and you'll start to see and feel real benefits. Squash is a hard and fast game but is very efficient at burning calories. If this is new to you, begin by playing gently. All these forms of exercise are brilliant for promoting shapely legs.

## Fruit & vegetables

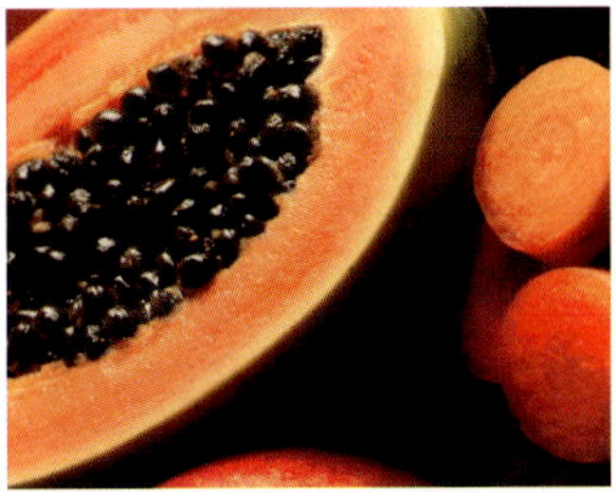

Aim for a minimum of 5 portions a day. A portion equals one medium-sized apple, a banana, 2 plums, a handful of cherry tomatoes, a large bowlful of salad, a 100 g slice of melon or 80 g cooked green vegetables.

Fruit and vegetables are referred to by nutritionists as 'nutrient-dense' foods. This means that they have a high amount of vitamins and minerals in comparison to the calories they contain. They are generally low in fat, rich in antioxidants, known to protect us from the most prevalent diseases, and a good source of fibre. Organic produce – which is grown without the use of chemical fertilizers and pesticides – is becoming increasingly popular and available at supermarkets, farmers' markets and greengrocers.

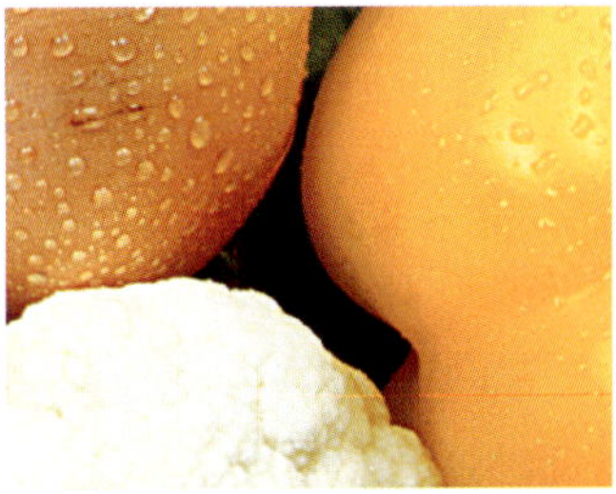

Try to eat a variety of fresh produce in a range of colours, from red and yellow peppers, oranges, carrots and berries to green leafy vegetables such as broccoli, cabbage, cauliflower and chard to provide your body with a powerful combination of beneficial phytochemicals and the antioxidants beta-carotene and vitamin C.

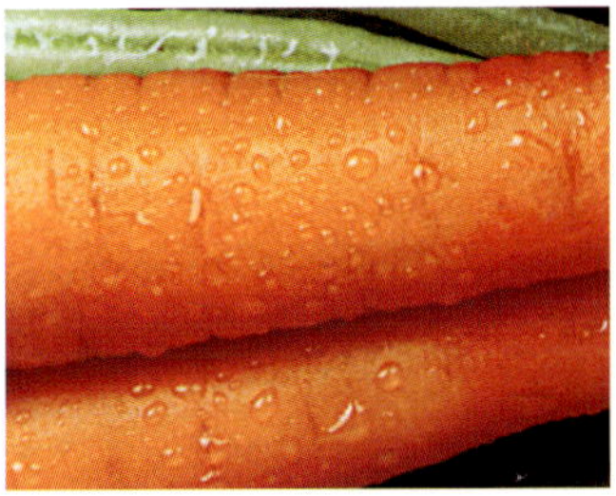

When cooking vegetables, steaming or stir-frying will retain more nutrients than boiling. Try to eat raw vegetables or salad at least once a day. Freshly squeezed juices have more nutrients than concentrated or long-life alternatives; a 150 ml glass will account for one of your 5 daily portions. Frozen fruit and vegetables can be just as high in vitamins as fresh, perhaps more so, if the fresh alternative has been stored for some time. Canned produce contains fewer nutrients, and you should opt for no sugar or salt varieties whenever possible.

**Aim to eat at least 5 portions of fruit and vegetables a day. Fresh, frozen, canned, dried and juiced all count.**

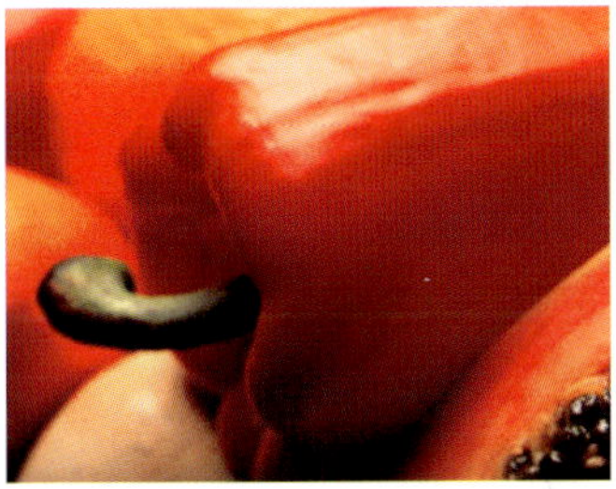

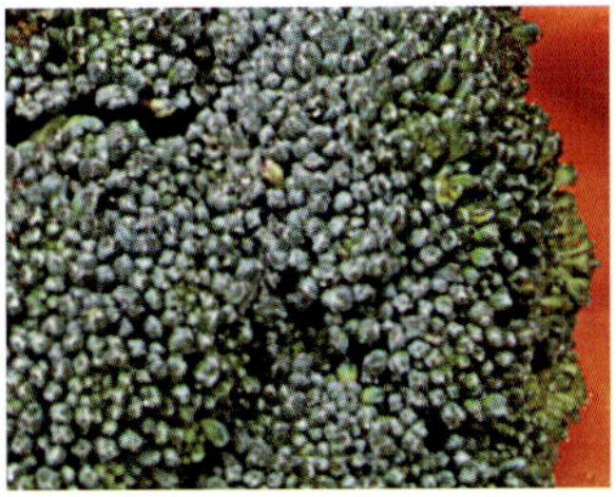

# Easy & enjoyable exercise ideas

## Cycling

Cycling is a great exercise for all the family. You could even on occasions turn it into a day's outing, stopping off for a picnic on the way. There are special off-road cycling areas around the country but if you are cycling on roads, make sure you know your Highway Code. You should wear a cycle helmet and at night, use lights and wear reflective clothing.

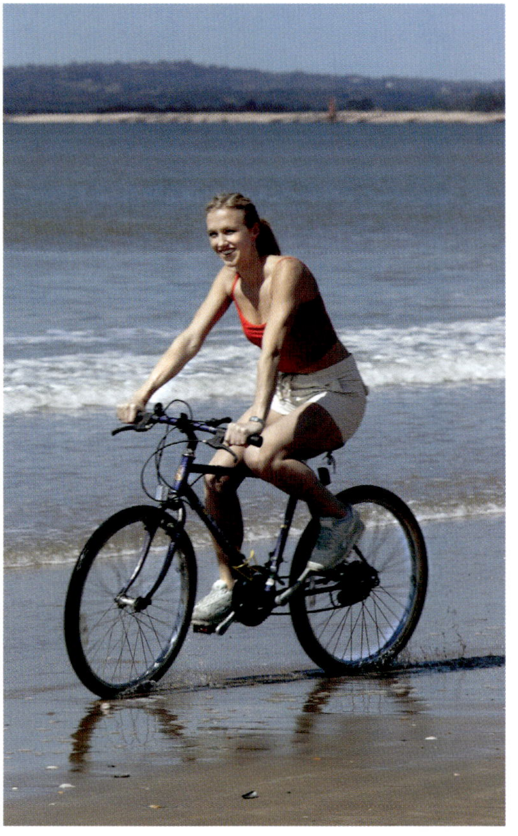

## Water aerobics

This is based on normal aerobic exercises, i.e. running, jogging and walking, but instead of it being done on land, the exercises are performed in water, generally at a local swimming pool. It is a perfect form of all-round exercise and, as your confidence grows, so you will find yourself able to move into a deeper section of the pool. Essentially the idea is to work the muscles against the resistance of the water while maintaining an upright stance throughout the exercise sequence. It is a great way of burning up calories efficiently.

## Power walking

How about taking up power walking? Not a gentle saunter around the park but a brisk walk, head and shoulders back, arms swinging, tummy held in and taking long determined strides. Not only will it encourage better posture, but power walking is also ideal for toning up the thighs, arms and legs. The more intense you make it, the more calories you will burn up. And when you are powering along, make sure that you take in deep breaths of fresh air.

**POWER WALKING CAN:**

- **help you shape up and at the same time burn approximately 350 calories an hour**
- **lower cholesterol**
- **regulate blood pressure**
- **relieve chronic pain**
- **help insomnia and infertility**
- **alleviate depression**

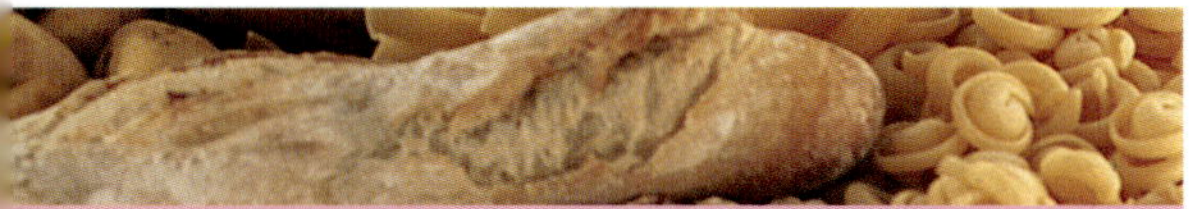

**Starchy carbohydrates (from bread, cereals and potatoes) should make up about one third of your daily diet, since they supply the body with the sustained energy that it needs to function effectively.**

### GI EXPLAINED

The GI Index (Glycaemic Index) is used to measure the rate at which all carbohydrate foods (including sugars and starches) are digested and converted to glucose to raise blood sugar levels and provide energy. Foods with a high GI are quickly broken down, giving a sudden rise in blood sugar and an immediate burst of energy. Foods with a low GI are absorbed more slowly, so you feel full for longer. Blood sugar levels are kept more constant providing long-term energy. The GI index is used by professionals to help treat diabetics but it's also now recognised that low-GI foods can help control hunger and appetite and are therefore good choices for 'slimmers'. Low-GI foods include all pulses, apples, grapefruit, dried apricots, green vegetables, natural yogurt and milk; medium-GI foods include pasta, oats, rice, pitta bread, boiled potatoes, sweetcorn and peas and examples of some high-GI foods are mashed potatoes, sugar, honey and popcorn.

## Bread, cereals & potatoes

This group includes cereals, bread, rice, noodles, pasta and potatoes, otherwise known as starchy (or complex) carbohydrate foods. Beans and lentils also provide starchy carbohydrates as well as being good sources of vegetable protein.

The more unrefined the better. Foods containing refined and processed grains and cereals not only contain fewer nutrients but lead to yo-yoing blood sugar levels, the effects of which are mood swings and variation in energy levels. Wholemeal is better than white, because these foods provide more fibre, B-group vitamins and minerals. Fibre helps to protect against digestive disorders and heart disease and comes in two forms: insoluble and soluble. Insoluble fibre helps to prevent constipation and bowel disorders by speeding up the passage of food through the large intestine. Whole wheat, brown rice and nuts are good sources of insoluble fibre. Soluble fibre, found mainly in beans, vegetables and oats, can reduce harmful blood cholesterol and help control blood sugar levels.

Carbohydrate foods are often accused of being fattening but it tends to be what you serve with them, such as butter, cheese or creamy sauces, that bumps up the calories and fat levels.

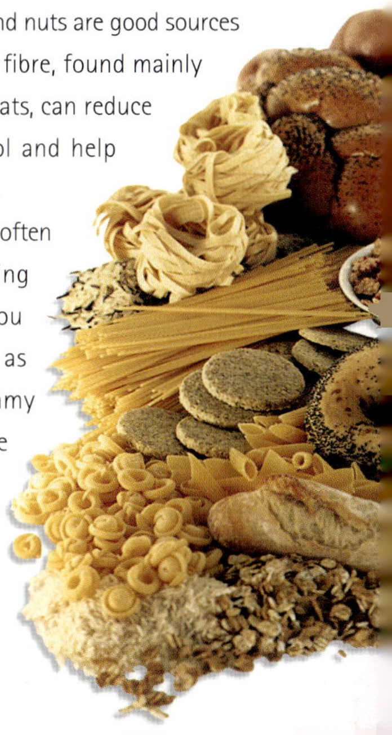

**Choose a wide variety of starchy carbohydrate foods. Unrefined (wholegrain types) are richer in nutrients and fibre.**

## Bouncing

Jogging and jumping on a trampoline is great aerobic exercise. It raises the heartbeat and increases lung capacity without putting unnecessary pressure on knee joints. You could join the local gym or invest in a mini-trampoline to use at home, indoors or out in the garden on days when the weather is good. All the family will be keen to use it!

## Kick boxing

This activity has become very popular with both men and women. Furthermore it:

- Helps lower body fat by toning the muscles
- Helps people to work out their stresses and frustrations
- Improves power, balance and overall agility
- Increases muscular endurance and strength
- Many women say that it enhances their self-confidence
- Tones and conditions the upper part of the body

Many local gyms run kick-boxing classes, so why not check them out?

**Exercise to energise. Keep those words firmly focused in your mind's eye – write them in large print on a piece of paper and pin it up in the kitchen or bathroom so that whenever you feel sluggish, you can remind yourself and keep yourself motivated.**

### HEALTH CHECK

- Before taking up any sport, check with your doctor if you are pregnant or have a medical condition
- Always warm up before starting and cool down slowly afterwards
- Never increase the intensity or length spent exercising if you feel any physical discomfort
- Make sure that you drink plenty of fluids while exercising
- Don't exercise if you feel unwell

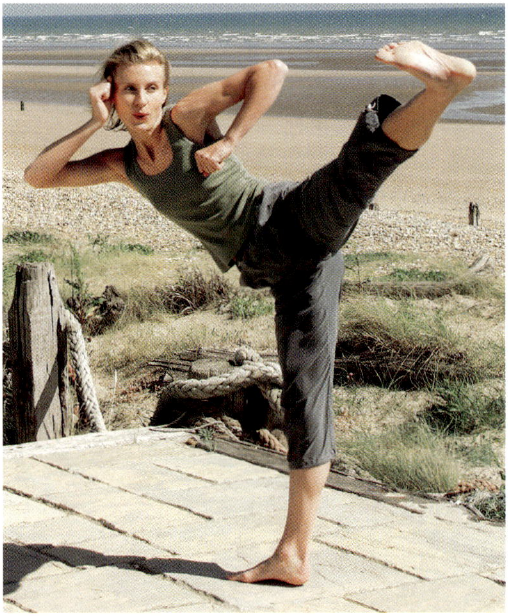

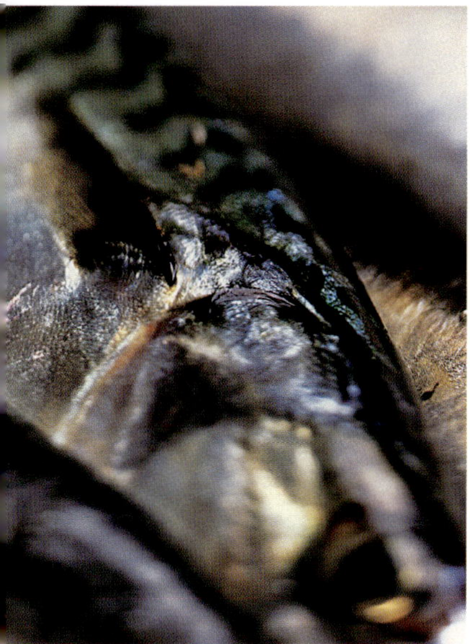

Oily fish contain essential fatty acids, which reduce your risk of heart disease and cancer.

Choose lean cuts of red meat and trim off any visible fat.

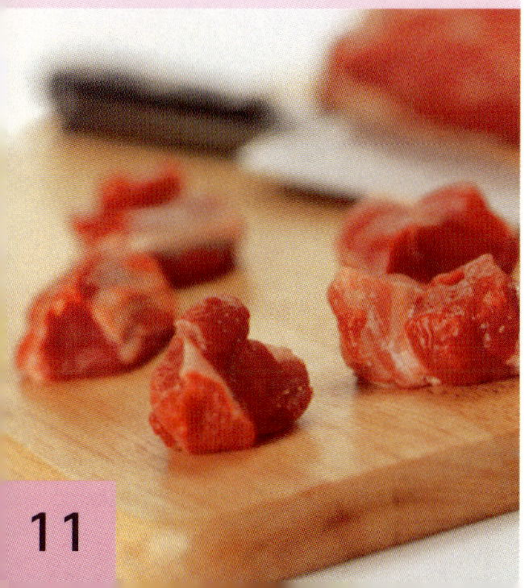

## Meat, fish & protein alternatives

This group includes meat, fish and poultry as well as eggs, nuts, pulses, seeds, Quorn and soya products such as tofu. They are all good sources of protein and should be eaten in moderate amounts daily, but try to eat a variety to ensure a good balance of amino acids. Protein foods are essential for growth, repair and maintenance in the body, and provide valuable amounts of iron, B-group vitamins, zinc, magnesium, vitamin E and fibre.

The body requires protein in relatively small amounts and in Western societies, we tend to eat more than we need. Limit red meat to about 3 servings a week, choose lean cuts and trim off any visible fat. Aim to eat fish at least twice a week and include at least one portion of oily fish such as herring, salmon, mackerel pilchards, sardines, trout or fresh tuna. These fish contain rich amounts of omega-3 fatty acids, which are thought to reduce the risk of heart disease. Limit your egg intake to 4 a week.

Since animal sources of protein can be high in fat, it is important to balance this with plant forms found in beans, peas and lentils. These are low in fat and high in fibre. Nuts and seeds are nutritious, are a good source of the essential fatty acid omega-6 but are relatively high in fat, so eat on a regular basis but in moderate amounts.

The high-protein diets that are currently fashionable may not be good for you in the long term. Studies have found a link between a high-protein diet and constipation, bowel disease and an increased risk of osteoporosis, since in excess protein encourages the excretion of calcium from the bones. Additionally, too much protein in the long term may affect kidney function

## Milk & dairy foods

Milk, cheese, yogurt and fromage frais provide valuable amounts of protein, calcium, some B-group vitamins, including $B_{12}$, $B_6$ and $B_2$, as well as vitamins A and D, essential for healthy teeth and bones and the release of energy from food. Eat these foods in moderation but opt for low or reduced-fat varieties, as dairy products, particularly hard cheese, can be high in saturated fat.

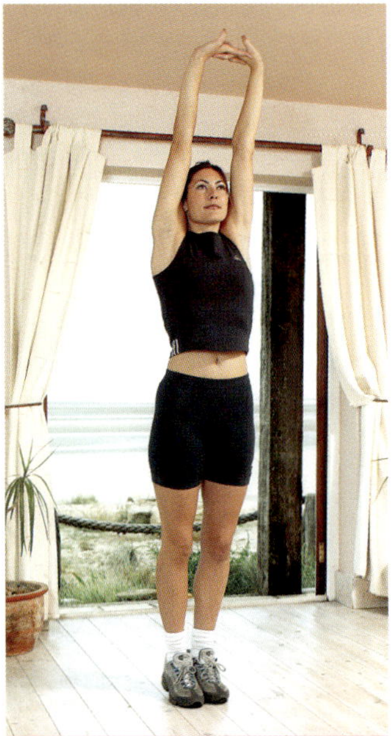

**MAKE SURE THAT EACH DAY YOU:**

- Kick start the body into action with an an energy shower each morning
- Do some stretching and flexing of the body at the start of each day
- Spend 30 minutes exercising
- Each day pamper yourself in some way
- Laugh heartily each day
- Aim to get a good night's sleep

## Move it to lose it

If apart from walking to the shops, you haven't exercised since the day you left school, then you are bound to feel a little apprehensive. But all the experts advocate a daily dose of physical activity to help us stay emotionally and physically fit. Exercise actually increases energy levels by releasing endorphins, which are the body's natural high hormones that make you feel great.

On the first day or so, just do some gentle exercise, walking to the shops instead of taking the car or getting the bus. Go for a swim or perhaps enrol at your local gym. If the concept of donning a leotard and taking up step aerobics fills you with horror or the mere mention of jogging causes an outbreak of athlete's foot, relax – there are plenty of other options.

The key advice is to participate in activities that you enjoy. It needs to be regular in order for it to be fully effective. Like most things in life, you only get out what you put in and apart from the physical benefits, becoming more active is a great way of socialising and meeting new people. Here are some ideas.

## Rise & stretch

A good stretch a day makes aches go away. Try it for yourself. Perform each movement slowly.

1. Link your fingers and raise them above your head until you feel the whole of your upper body stretch.
2. Still keeping your fingers linked, stretch your arms out in front at the same time stretching your back.
3. Place your arms behind you, still with your fingers linked, and as you stretch feel the pull across your chest.
4. Drop your left ear down to your left shoulder, stretching out the muscles of the neck and shoulders, then do the same on the other side.
5. To stretch the back of your neck, drop your chin down to your chest.

Use skimmed or semi-skimmed milk rather than whole milk in drinks, on cereals and for cooking. Semi-skimmed (half-fat) milk tastes like whole (full-fat) milk but has had the cream poured off. Skimmed milk has had almost all of the fat removed and has a 'thinner' taste. Both skimmed and semi-skimmed have as much protein and in fact slightly more calcium than whole milk, although the fat-soluble vitamins A and D are reduced, but with less fat and fewer calories make a healthier and lighter choice.

Soya, oat or rice milks make good alternatives to cow's milk and are often fortified to provide a good source of calcium. Organic dairy products are also becoming more widely available and make good, healthy choices as they are free from antibiotic residues, growth hormones and agrochemicals.

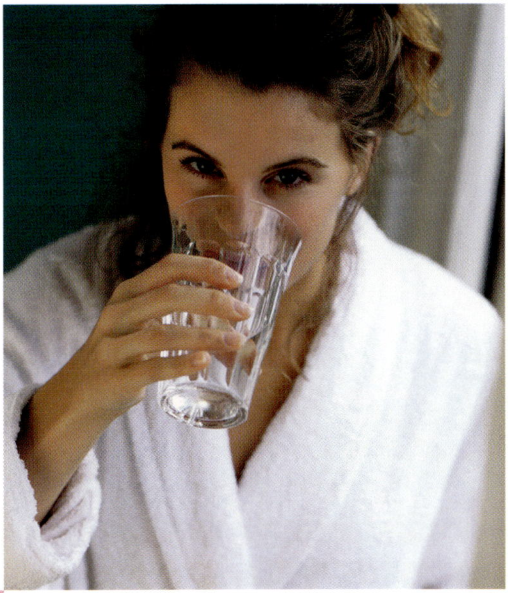

**Low or reduced-fat dairy products are the healthiest option. Natural live bio yogurt helps to maintain a healthy intestinal environment.**

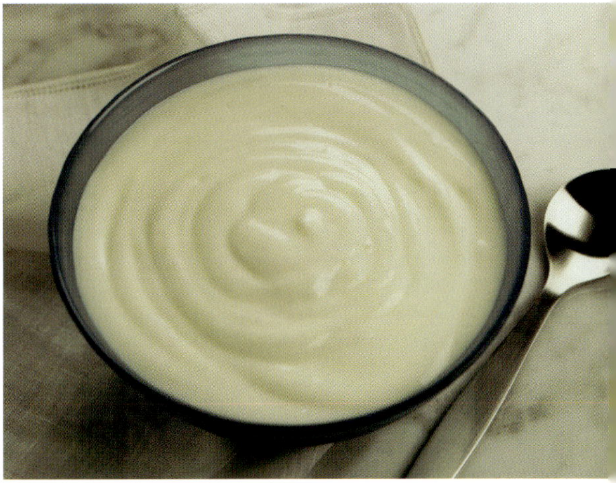

## Water

Water plays a vital role in maintaining good health and flushes out toxins and waste products. It also promotes good digestion, improves vitality and the health of your skin and drinking plenty of water will reduce the risk of bladder infections, constipation and headaches. It's best to choose filtered or natural mineral water to achieve the desired daily amount. Coffee, tea and fizzy drinks contain caffeine, which has a diuretic effect, so they actually dehydrate the body. Herbal or rooibos (red) tea are healthy, caffeine-free alternatives.

**Aim to drink 6–8 glasses (1.7–2 litres/ 3–3$^{1}/_{5}$ pints) of water a day.**

# Putting exercise into action

## Ways of getting started

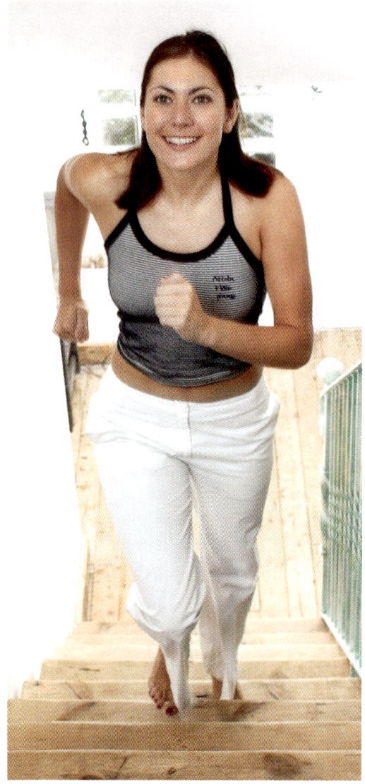

You don't have to join a gym to get fit. There are many things you can do that you may not have considered to be exercise that are easily incorporated into your life: walk up the stairs instead of taking the lift, walk or cycle to work, take the dog for regular walks, take the children to play in the park at the weekend and join in (and this will benefit the whole family), or simply put on some music and dance around the living room.

To start exercising, aim to do 15–20 minutes at least three times a week. Follow an exercise routine you enjoy, such as swimming, walking or cycling, because you are then much more likely to stick to it. As your body gets stronger you should increase the length and intensity of the exercise, but always be aware of how your body is feeling during and after exercise. If you feel exhausted, take more rest until your vitality increases. Build up gradually, especially if you have not exercised for a while.

Once you have built up your strength and energy levels you can move on to regular cardiovascular exercise. This enhances detoxing and increases the oxygen uptake in your body. Cycling, running, swimming, tennis, yoga and aerobics are all suitable. Aim to exercise for at least half an hour five times a week.

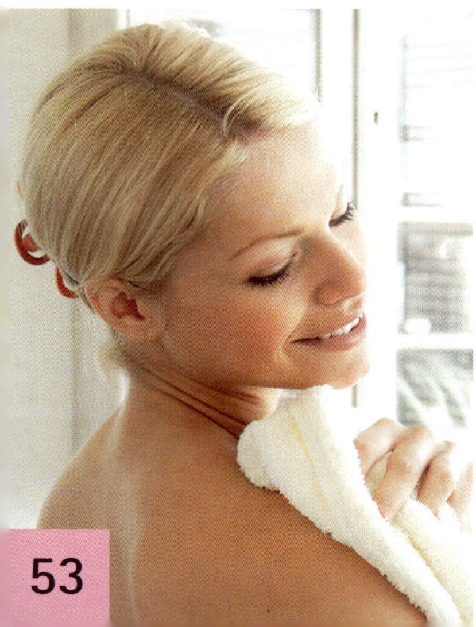

## Energy shower

There is nothing like an early morning energy shower to kick-start the body into action, so first thing each morning jump into the shower and, if you feel brave enough, when you are about ready to come out, turn the cold tap full on for a few minutes.

After showering, invigorate your body and boost circulation by slapping yourself all over. Using the flats of your hands and slap from toes to hip, wrist to shoulder and all over your chest, shoulders and torso before rubbing dry with a towel.

# What to avoid

## Fats

A small amount of fat in the diet is essential for good health and to make foods taste pleasant to eat. However we tend to eat far more fat than we need and this is linked with a higher risk of heart disease as well as frequently causing an excess gain in weight. Fats provide a concentrated source of energy and more than twice the calories provided by proteins or carbohydrates.

There are two main types of fat: saturated and unsaturated. Unsaturated fats come in two forms, monounsaturated and polyunsaturated and are found in oily fish, vegetable oils, nuts and seeds. They help lower cholesterol levels in the blood and reduce fatty deposits furring up the arteries, thereby helping to prevent the risk of blood clots, strokes and heart disease. Saturated fats, however, found mainly in animal products, should be kept to a minimum because they increase cholesterol in the blood, which increases the risk of heart disease. Choose lean cuts of red meat and trim visible fat, skin poultry, eat oil-rich fish and opt for low or reduced-fat dairy products. There are also saturated fats hidden in chocolate, biscuits, cakes, pastry and crisps and although you can often buy lower-fat versions of many of these foods, they should be restricted, especially if you are trying to lose weight.

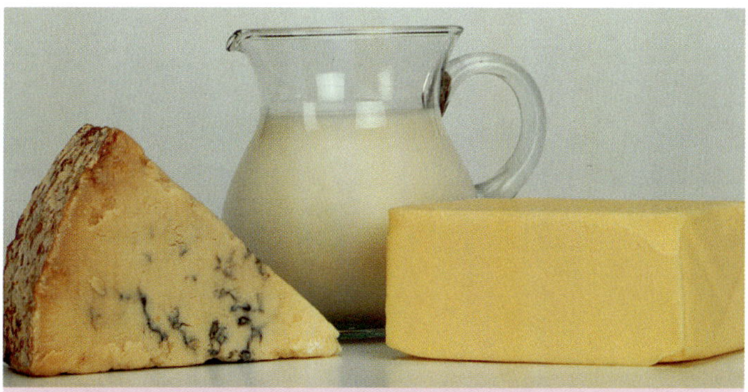

Dairy products, especially hard cheeses like Cheddar and Stilton, are high in saturated fat, so limit your intake. Choose semi-skimmed milk.

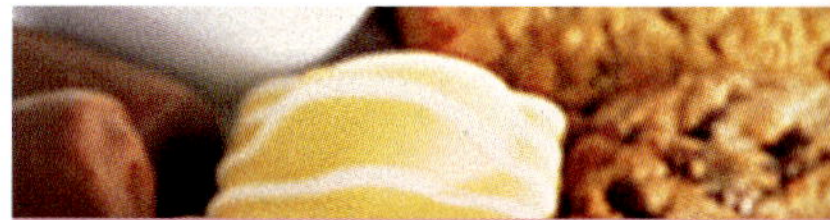

**Deciding which foods to cut back on is just as crucial as what you choose to include in your diet. Foods high in sugar, fat and salt provide the body with negligible nutrients and can do more harm than good.**

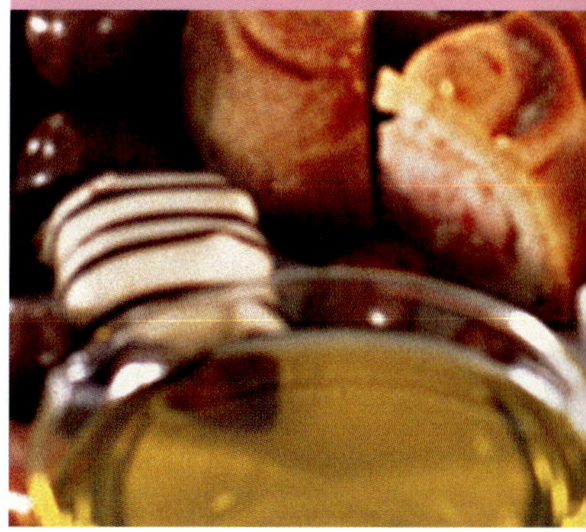

Margarine, once hailed as the healthy alternative to butter, is often laden with additives, preservatives and hydrogenated or trans fats, which have been found to be possibly more harmful to your health than saturates. This type of fat is also found in processed foods. Check labels and try to avoid products that include hydrogenated fats/oils in the ingredients list.

# Putting exercise into action

Regular exercise is an essential part of any healthy dieting regime. Not only will it help to burn up calories and stored body fat but it will increase your metabolism and improve muscle tone. Regular gentle exercise also builds up your stamina, flexibility and strength, and is invaluable in maintaining a healthy body, mind and spirit. Repetitive exercise such as swimming, walking or running is also a golden opportunity for you to enjoy self-reflection, mental relaxation and meditation.

## KEY BENEFITS OF EXERCISE

- Speeds up metabolism
- Helps control cholesterol and burns fat
- Muscular movement enables your body's systems to work more efficiently, removing toxins
- Increases muscle strength, which can help to prevent back pain
- Makes your body more efficient at using oxygen
- Promotes deep breathing, which is key to relaxation
- Makes you physically tired and aids sleep
- Improves joint mobility and stability, which can help to keep you active and independent in later life
- Improves circulation
- Causes the release of the body's natural painkillers, endorphins, which reduce anxiety and leave you feeling relaxed and in a better mood
- Releases adrenalin, thus reducing stress
- Improves self-esteem
- Strengthens the heart and helps reduce blood pressure
- Increases your body's ability to fight off infection
- Helps keep bones strong and healthy
- Meditative exercise such as t'ai chi help you focus your mind and improve co-ordination

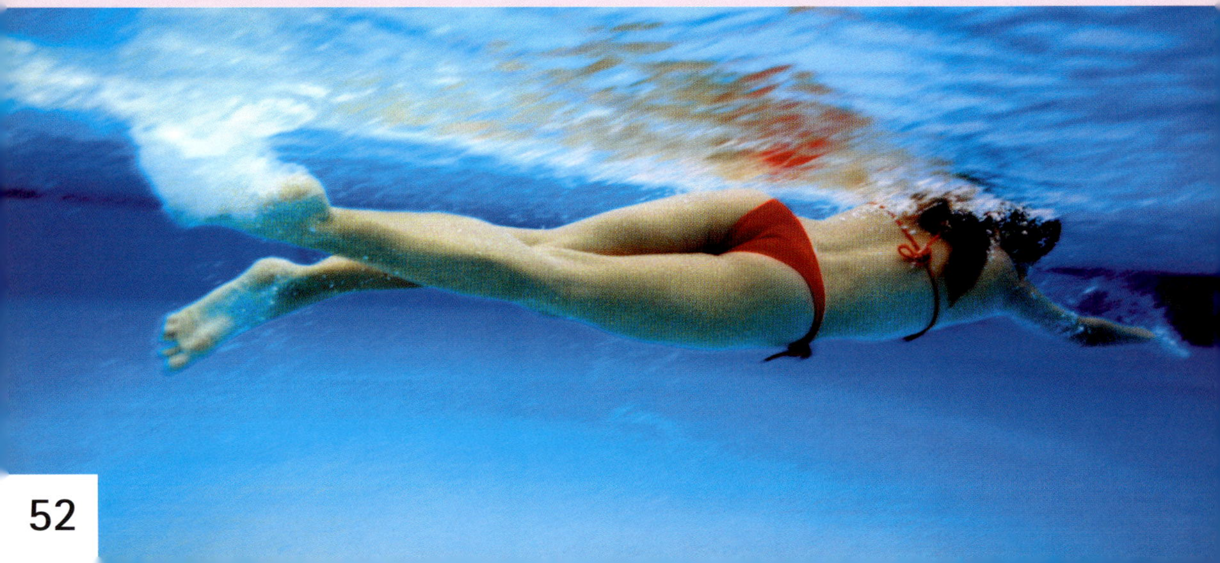

**Moderation is the key. There's no need to deny yourself completely but try to limit sweet foods and to enjoy them as occasional treats. When shopping, look out for sucrose, fructose, glucose, maltose, corn syrup, invert sugar and dextrose on food labels, which are basically sugar by another name.**

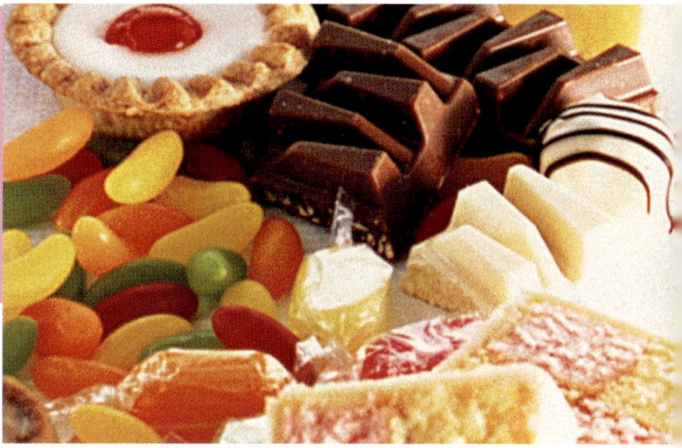

## Sugar

Refined sugars and those found in processed foods, including biscuits, sweets, cakes, puddings and fizzy drinks, have little or no nutritional value. They simply provide 'empty' calories and if you are trying to lose weight, cutting back on sugar is one of the easiest ways to cut calories without losing nutrients. You do not need sugar for energy – you get energy from all the other foods you eat.

Eating a sugary food also only gives a temporary surge in energy, which is promptly followed by a slump. It is this fluctuation in blood sugar levels that leads to an inconsistent supply of energy to the brain, leading to poor concentration, mood swings, brain 'fug' and tiredness. Consequently, you soon feel the need for another quick energy fix to boost your energy back up again. Not only does this yo-yo effect in blood sugar play havoc with your energy levels and encourage snacking on high calorific foods, but eating too much sugar is a major cause of tooth decay.

Low-sugar foods sweetened with artificial sweeteners, such as saccharin and aspartame, do not contribute to tooth decay and are virtually calorie-free but they do perpetuate a sweet tooth. They are helpful when dieting but as a longer term goal, it's better to try and gradually wean yourself off sweet-tasting foods and drinks.

## Salt

We are all eating too much salt. The average adult consumption is 9.5g of salt a day, but experts recommend no more than 6g (equivalent to a teaspoonful). There are about 2.5g of sodium in 6g of salt and it's the sodium that can cause health problems. Excess salt is a major cause of high blood pressure, which leads to strokes and heart attacks. Too much salt in the diet has also been linked to fluid retention and kidney stones.

Most of the salt we eat comes from processed foods, which also tend to be high in fat and calories. Crisps, crackers, salted nuts, stock cubes, packet soups and cheese are obvious culprits but, surprisingly, a bowl of cornflakes is higher in salt than a bag of crisps! Other processed foods that contain high amounts of salt include biscuits, baked beans and bread. The salt we need is supplied in adequate amounts in natural foods such as meat, fish and vegetables. So, as well as cutting back on processed foods and salty snacks, choose foods with less added salt, use less salt in cooking and do not add salt at the table.

# Eating out

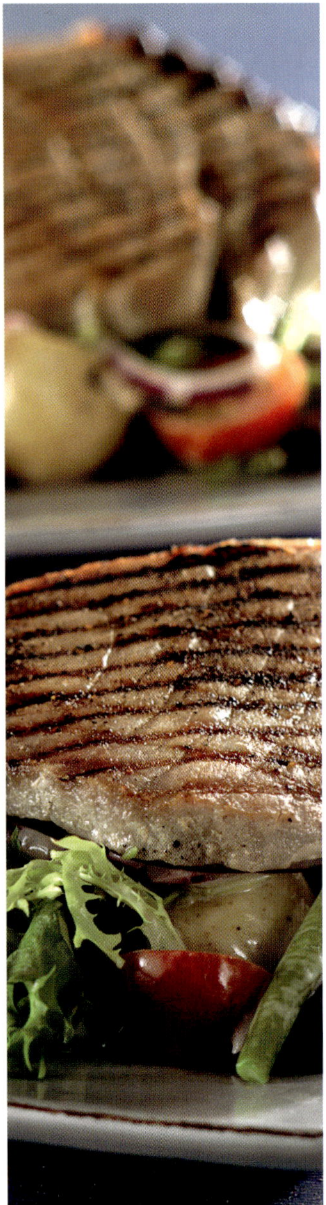

- Trim fat from steak and remove skin from poultry.
- You can enjoy a roast but go steady on the roast potatoes and Yorkshire pudding and fill your plate with plenty of vegetables.
- Grilled kebabs in pitta bread with salad make a good healthy choice.
- Tandoori or tikka dishes are prepared from marinated foods that are then oven-baked. Serve with a salad, yogurt raita and naan bread, chapattis or plain boiled rice.
- Pasta is a good starchy carbohydrate and satisfying to eat but watch out for rich sauces that tend to be high in fat and calories. Opt for tomato and seafood sauces and resist anything creamy or very cheesy.
- Pizza too can be a healthy choice but don't choose one that's loaded with cheese or pepperoni, which are both high in fat. Chicken, ham and pineapple, seafood or vegetable toppings are better choices. You can have a thin or thick crust but avoid stuffed crust.
- It's best to avoid chips or mashed potato. Boiled new potatoes or a small jacket potato are better choices.
- Avoid salads already coated with dressing. If you like a dressing, ask for it separately to drizzle lightly yourself.
- Go for plain cooked vegetables.
- Many desserts, such as gateâux, pastries and anything with cream will be high in fat. Go for a fruity choice or if you can't resist, a small portion of something wicked!
- Take your time eating giving your food a chance to reach your stomach and allow you to feel pleasantly satisfied rather than uncomfortably bloated. Don't feel that you have to finish every last morsel that's on your plate. If you've had enough, leave the rest.
- Be adventurous and try new dishes. A healthy diet means enjoying plenty of variety and should never be boring. So use the occasion to try some thing you haven't had before or something you wouldn't cook at home.

Bon appetit!

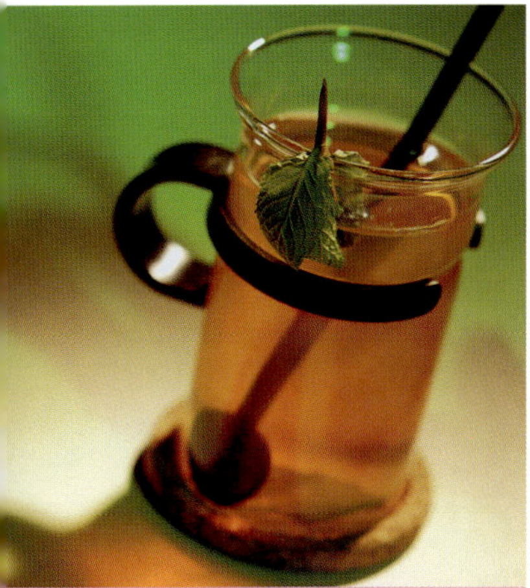

Herb teas are naturally caffeine-free.

## Caffeine

Caffeine is a stimulant, which means it helps to keep us alert and awake. If drunk in excess (over 8 cups a day), however, it can lead to the jitters, shakes, headaches, an irregular heartbeat and stomach upsets. It is also a diuretic, causing dehydration in the body. Those at risk of osteoporosis should pay special attention to their caffeine intake, since it increases the excretion of calcium in the urine. It also inhibits the absorption of vitamins and minerals from the gut.

Coffee contains about 40 per cent more caffeine than tea and chocolate. Strong continental brands, in particular, are more likely to have noticeable side effects. Fizzy drinks, like cola, also contain caffeine. Try to limit yourself to no more than three caffeine drinks a day. Herbal teas and coffee alternatives are healthier options.

## Alchohol

Alcohol, in moderation, can be included in your diet but remember that it is high in calories and contains little nutrient value, so if you are trying to lose weight, restrict yourself to an occasional tipple.

Wine or spirits are generally better choices as beer and lager tend to be drunk in larger measures. Spirits can be served with sugar-free mixers or tomato juice, which provides powerful lycopene, a beneficial antioxidant. Red wine also contains antioxidants, known as flavonols, that are good for your heart and circulation since they help to make the blood less prone to clotting and protect against coronary heart disease. Antioxidants also help to mop up harmful free radicals in the body thus reducing cell damage known to cause cancer. Go for quality rather than quantity and treat yourself to a glass of really good wine rather than several glasses of plonk! A white wine spritzer, mixed with half quantity sparkling mineral water, also makes a good low-calorie choice.

For good general health, alcohol should be treated with respect. Women should not exceed 14 units of alcohol a week, men 21 units. Avoid binge drinking and spread your intake throughout the week, keeping two consecutive days completely alcohol-free.

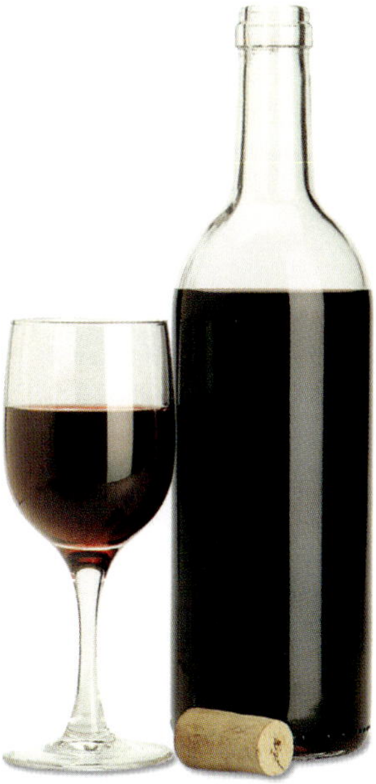

You can enjoy a favourite tipple on your diet but alcohol is high in calories so this should be an occasional treat.

# Eating out

No need to avoid going out to restaurants when dieting. Just think before ordering, as it's all too easy to be tempted by a menu and over indulge. However, if you really fancy that slice of chocolate gâteau or some other treat, don't spoil the occasion by denying yourself. So often, diets fail because they're too strict and rule out certain foods. One thing you can guarantee is that imposing a ban on a particular food will ensure that you crave it constantly! Dieting by eating healthily is not about denial but about making sensible food choices, eating a wide variety of foods and allowing yourself those yummy extras as occasional treats. Remember, it's only one meal and going slightly over the top now and again won't make a huge difference to your overall intake, if you generally eat moderately. Besides, you can always work off those extra calories with a bit more exercise.

## Tips

- Order first so you won't instantly want what other people have ordered.
- Generally speaking, our eyes are bigger than our stomachs so try to order a little less than you think you could eat. Ask yourself, do you really need 3 courses plus a bread roll and butter, plus chocolates with coffee?  Be honest and think before 'pigging out'. You'll only regret it later!
- Order a large bottle of mineral water for the table to avoid drinking too much alcohol. Drinking water will also help take the edge off your appetite.
- Grilled, steamed, stir-fried or baked dishes are generally good choices but try to avoid anything deep-fried, battered, crumbed, prepared in pastry or in a rich creamy sauce.

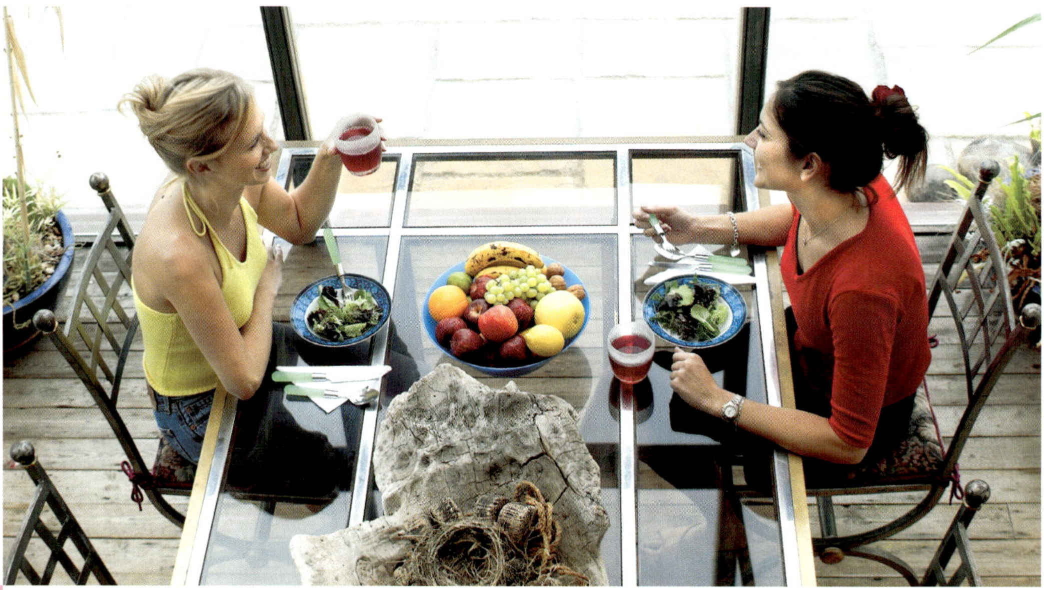

## 3 WEEK MEAL PLANNER

The following pages contain suggested menus that are carefully planned to help you make healthy food choices. There are no weights included because by choosing the right kinds of foods, your appetite will naturally control how much you eat. The menus are designed to be flexible so you can mix and match the ideas to suit your personal taste and to fit in with your lifestyle. Weekday lunches are ideas that can be easily packed up to take to work but if you prefer, you can swap the lunch with the dinner. What's important is that you include plenty of variety and don't skip meals so that your appetite is satisfied and there's less risk from temptation to nibble between meals. Combine this eating plan with regular exercise and after just 3 weeks, you should be looking and feeling trimmer and fitter. Stick to the guidelines and you'll find it easy to reach and maintain the size and figure you want.

## Guidelines

- Eat 3 meals a day - breakfast, lunch and dinner. Don't skip meals and in particular, make time for breakfast to get your day off to a really healthy start.

- Eat a wide variety of different foods. This will help ensure your diet includes all the nutrients needed for good health.

- Go for lean meat, fish and poultry, starchy carbohydrates like bread, rice, pasta and potatoes and aim for at least 5 portions of fruit and vegetables daily. Wholegrain cereals, like wholemeal bread, brown rice and oats are particularly satisfying to eat and like fruit, vegetables and pulses are good sources of fibre needed for a healthy digestion.

- Cut down on high-fat and sugary foods and unnecessary snacks between meals. For weak moments, choose a satisfying, low-fat snack (see ideas on page 42).

- You can have up to 300 ml / ½ pint semi-skimmed milk each day for hot drinks or try refreshing herbal teas, hot lemon or blackcurrant or Bovril as alternatives.

- You can also have one treat daily (see ideas on page 42). These are not essential (and can be omitted) but include many of the foods and drinks we love and by not banning them completely, it can be easier to stick to a diet. However be warned, it's these types of foods that can so easily bump up your calorie intake, making flab more difficult to shift, so keep such treats to a minimum. Keeping active will help to burn these extra calories.

- Drink plenty of water – aim for 6 – 8 glasses daily. Add ice and a slice of lemon or if you're not keen on plain water, add a splash of fruit juice or cordial to sparkling mineral water.

EGGS

The ultimate convenience food so always keep a box in the fridge for a quick meal.

CHEESE

Go for mature-flavoured cheeses, like Parmesan, Stilton or mature Cheddar, so you only need use a little for a lot of flavour. Cheeses like Brie, camembert and Edam are lower in fat and calories than hard cheeses. Low-fat soft cheeses are good for dips and spreads.

SPREADS

Low or reduced-fat spreads are one option. If you use margarine, choose one labelled 'high in polyunsaturates' or 'high in monounsaturates'. Avoid those that contain hydrogenated oils or trans fats. A small amount of butter is fine for when the flavour really counts. Remember that margarines contain the same amount of fat and calories as butter – it's just the type of fat that is different - so spread it thinly.

NUTS & SEEDS

Nourishing for sprinkling and as a healthy nibble. Buy in small quantities and store in an air-tight tin, in the dark as they can become rancid.

SALAD DRESSINGS

You can buy low-fat dressings, and reduced-fat mayonnaise or light dressings based on yogurt or tomato juice. Alternatively a small amount of French dressing, made with olive oil, can be lightly tossed into a salad.

CANNED FOODS

Canned pulses are an economical, low-fat, nutritious food and are useful for adding to soups, casseroles and salads. Go for varieties canned in water rather than brine and baked beans with reduced-sugar and salt. Canned fish is also a good healthy buy. Choose ones canned in spring water or tomato sauce.

FROZEN FOODS

Fruits and vegetables make convenient and healthy alternatives and help add greater variety to your diet.

PACKAGED FOODS

Check labels and avoid buying those with high amounts of sugar, saturated and hydrogenated (trans) fats, salt (sodium) and artificial additives. Don't be taken in by terms like 'natural', 'country' or 'traditional' as they mean little when used on processed foods.

## USEFUL STORE-CUPBOARD BASICS

Tomato puree • Worcestershire, soy, cranberry, pesto and horseradish sauce • Mustard • Redcurrant jelly • Mayonnaise (reduced fat) • Canned oily fish • Fruit (in juice) • Tomatoes • Sweetcorn • Pasta, pulses and rice (various) • Wholegrain cereals • Sugar-free muesli and porridge oats • Spreads – honey, peanut butter, yeast extract • Dried fruits • Unsalted nuts and seeds • Stock cubes • Herbs and spices • Olive oil • Vegetable oil (groundnut or sunflower) • Wine/cider vinegar • Plain flour and cornflour

Week one

| | BREAKFAST | LUNCH | DINNER |
|---|---|---|---|
| MONDAY | Sugar-free muesli with skimmed or semi-skimmed milk. If liked, top with yogurt and sliced strawberries. Glass of freshly squeezed orange juice or unsweetened fruit juice. | Pasta salad made with wholewheat pasta shapes, drained and flaked, canned tuna or salmon, sweetcorn, chopped cucumber and spring onions lightly tossed with reduced-fat mayonnaise, flavoured with a little lemon zest. Apple or handful of grapes. | Chicken and vegetable stir-fry. Use a selection of fresh vegetables such as strips of red pepper, carrots and bean sprouts and toss over a high heat with strips of chicken breast. Add your favourite stir-fry sauce and serve with boiled rice. |
| TUESDAY | Half a pink grapefruit, sweetened with 1 tsp honey/sugar (optional). Thick slice of wholemeal toast spread with peanut butter. | Hummus (see page 23) with vegetable crudités and wholemeal pitta bread. Pear or nectarine. | Honey-glazed salmon (see page 34) served with rice or couscous and lightly steamed broccoli or other fresh green vegetable. |
| WEDNESDAY | Greek-style or vanilla yogurt (low-fat) topped with fresh fruit, such as sliced banana and raspberries and sprinkled with 2 tbsp sugar-free muesli or 1 tbsp sunflower and pumpkin seeds or chopped nuts. | Tomato & courgette soup (see page 24) or other non-creamy, vegetable soup with hunk of wholemeal or multigrain bread (unbuttered). If liked, sprinkle a little grated cheese on top of the soup. | Chilli con carne (see page 35) with reduced-fat garlic bread (2 slices) and Sweetcorn & tomato salsa (see page 30). |
| THURSDAY | Boiled egg with wholemeal toast, thinly spread with yeast extract. Glass of unsweetened fruit juice. | Jacket potato topped with cottage cheese and prawns. Fruit salad made with sliced kiwi fruit, grapes and cubes of melon, moistened with unsweetened fruit juice. | Mushroom risotto served with lightly cooked spinach and a tomato and chive salad, lightly drizzled with French dressing. |

# Good food shopping guide

## BREAD & CEREALS

Choose wholemeal varieties wherever possible such as wholemeal bread (or Granary or multi-grain), whole-wheat pasta and brown rice. Dark rye bread makes a good alternative to wheat loaves. Breakfast cereals are also a good source of starchy carbohydrate and fibre. Go for ones with wholegrain ingredients and that are low in salt and added sugar. Porridge oats and sugar-free muesli are good choices.

## MEAT

Choose lean cuts of meat, such as extra-lean mince and super-trimmed (preferably reduced-salt) bacon. Venison makes a healthy, low-fat choice. Opt for good quality sausages and burgers with a high meat content and minimum amount of fat and fillers.

## FRESH HERBS

Buy freely. They're brilliant for adding flavour to all kinds of dishes so you can use less salt for seasoning.

## FISH

Buy frequently (fresh, frozen or canned), aiming for 2-3 fish meals a week. Good choices of oily fish, rich in omega-3 fatty acids, include salmon, mackerel, sardines, herring, trout and fresh tuna. Choose fish without batter or breadcrumbs or dishes prepared in rich, creamy sauces.

## FRUIT & VEGETABLES

Fill up your trolley with lots of these. Whenever possible buy organic, seasonal and local produce which is usually fresher and more nutritious as it hasn't been transported thousands of miles or kept in cold storage. Buy to eat on a regular basis rather than storing for long periods.

## MILK & YOGURT

Buy skimmed or semi-skimmed milk, low-fat yogurts and fromage frais. Soya milk is another healthy choice. Watch out for added sugar in fruit yogurts.

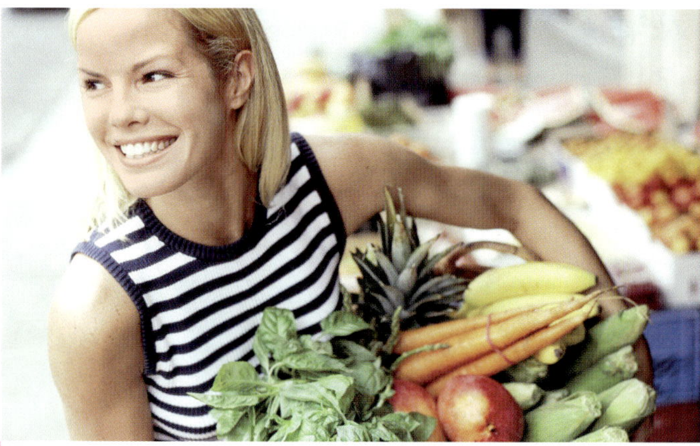

**Buy fresh foods from shops with a high turnover of goods. Farmer's markets or direct from a farm is a good way to source fresh produce – it can also be a lot cheaper. Shop with a list and don't shop when hungry so you're less likely to be tempted by impulse buys that may not be the healthiest choices.**

Week one

| | BREAKFAST | LUNCH | DINNER |
|---|---|---|---|
| FRIDAY | Peach & strawberry smoothie. Place 1 chopped peach and 115g (4oz) strawberries in a blender or food processor with 150ml (5 fl oz) each of semi-skimmed milk and natural low-fat yogurt. Blend until smooth. | Baguette (unbuttered) spread with cranberry sauce and filled with sliced brie and rocket. | Stuffed vegetables (see page 38). Crème caramel with sliced oranges. |
| SATURDAY | Toasted bagel or muffin topped with scrambled egg and mushrooms. Whisk eggs with a little semi-skimmed milk and freshly ground black pepper then cook gently in a non-stick pan with just a small knob of butter or in the microwave, until softly set. Add sliced button mushrooms, first microwaved in a little water. | Chickpea & tomato salad (see page 27) with cubes of feta or grilled smoked tofu or goat's cheese tossed in. Large slice of watermelon | Grilled kebabs. Make with cubes of chicken, lean pork or lamb or monkfish, marinated in a herb and garlic flavoured olive oil then threaded on to skewers with chunks of mixed peppers and wedges of red onions. Serve in warm flat bread with a leafy salad, drizzled with a tomato or yogurt dressing. |
| SUNDAY | Bacon and tomato butty. Fill a hunk of French bread or ciabatta (unbuttered) with grilled, lean back bacon and thickly sliced tomatoes. Add a little mustard, ketchup or brown sauce if liked | Roast chicken or turkey (skinned) served with mixed root mash (potatoes and swede mashed with low-fat, natural fromage frais and snipped chives), carrots and lightly steamed or stir-fried cabbage, redcurrant jelly or cranberry sauce. Raspberry & oat crunch (see page 40). | Grilled vegetable soup (see page 25) with toasted pitta pizzas. Spread wholemeal pittas with sun-dried tomato pureé, sprinkle with dried oregano and a little grated mozzarella then grill until bubbling. Cut into thick strips. |

## FOOD PREPARATION

**It's not just what you eat, but how you prepare and cook it that counts. The main culprit is fat, so low-fat cooking will not only help you to lose weight but will also encourage long-term healthy eating habits. Cutting back on sugary foods, such as cakes, biscuits, puddings and sweets, will also cut unnecessary calories, although a little of what you fancy occasionally won't do any harm.**

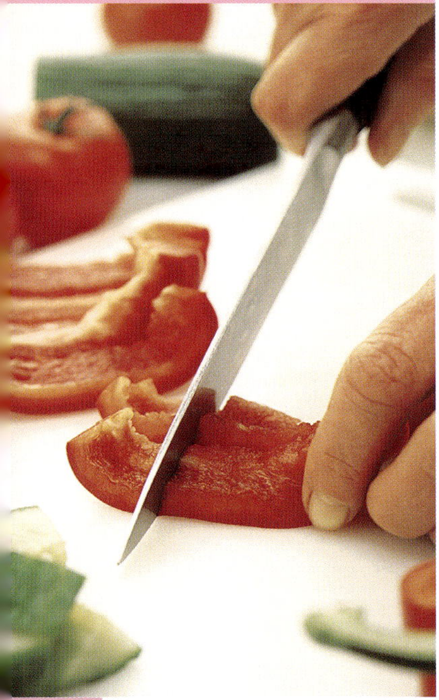

- Pastry dishes are high in fat, especially if made with puff pastry. Filo pastry, lightly brushed with oil between the layers, is the best option for lighter results.
- Think twice before putting that knob of butter on your vegetables. Sprinkle with freshly ground black pepper or toss with chopped, fresh herbs instead.
- You can treat yourself to chips occasionally but these should be thick cut and oven baked or grilled. Potato wedges make a healthier alternative. Scrub potatoes (leaving skins on), cut into thick wedges then place on a non-stick baking sheet and lightly brush with a little oil. Sprinkle with a spicy seasoning then bake until golden and tender.
- Roast potatoes can also be enjoyed occasionally (say once a week) but don't cook them in deep oil. Cut potatoes into large chunks, par-boil and drain well then place in a non-stick tin, brush with a little oil and roast in a hot oven until golden and crispy. Drain on kitchen paper before serving.
- Lighten mayonnaise with half quantity low-fat yogurt for salad dressings.

## CUT BACK ON SUGAR

- If you have a sweet tooth, try to gradually wean yourself off sugar by beginning to add a little less. Over time, you'll start to lose your liking for sugar and prefer foods that taste less sweet. Less sugar means you taste more flavour from the food itself.
- For fruit salads, use an unsweetened fruit juice rather than making a sweet, sugar syrup.
- Try halving the sugar you use in recipes. It works for most things except meringues, ice-cream and cakes.
- Use reduced-sugar jams and marmalades. Honey has the same calorie value as sugar and only a minute amount of nutrients, so use it with caution.
- If you like a pudding sometimes, choose one based on fruit. Not only is fruit healthy to eat but it is naturally sweet, so there's less need for added sugar.

## Week two

| | BREAKFAST | LUNCH | DINNER |
| --- | --- | --- | --- |
| MONDAY | Wholegrain cereal or sugar-free muesli with semi-skimmed milk. Glass of unsweetened orange or grapefruit juice. | Egg and watercress sandwich. Blend chopped hard-boiled egg with a little reduced-fat mayonnaise and season with freshly ground black pepper then spread on thickly sliced multigrain or rye bread. Cherry tomatoes and satsuma. | Grilled sausages with Ratatouille (see page 33) and potato wedges or thick cut oven chips. |
| TUESDAY | Mixed berry smoothie. Blend 115g (4oz) fruits of the forest with 150ml (5 fl oz) each semi-skimmed milk and reduced-fat Greek-style yogurt. | Chicken, avocado & rocket wrap (see page 32). Handful of dried apricots. | Penne with broccoli, peppers & pine nuts (see page 36). |
| WEDNESDAY | Beans on toast. Choose reduced-sugar baked beans and serve on thickly sliced, toasted wholemeal or multigrain bread. Glass of cran-berry juice. | Roast beef and salad sandwich. Thinly spread thickly sliced bread with butter and horseradish then pack with salad and sliced, lean roast beef. Low-fat fruit yogurt. | Spanish omelette (see page 37) served with a tomato and red onion side salad drizzled with a little French dressing. Thick slice of melon. |
| THURSDAY | Sliced banana stirred into natural low-fat yogurt, sprinkled with sugar-free muesli and blueberries | Lentil & carrot soup (see page 26) or other vegetable soup (not creamy). Serve with soda bread or a wholemeal roll (unbut-tered). | Grilled chicken (skinned) served with Watercress, orange & walnut salad (see page 28). |

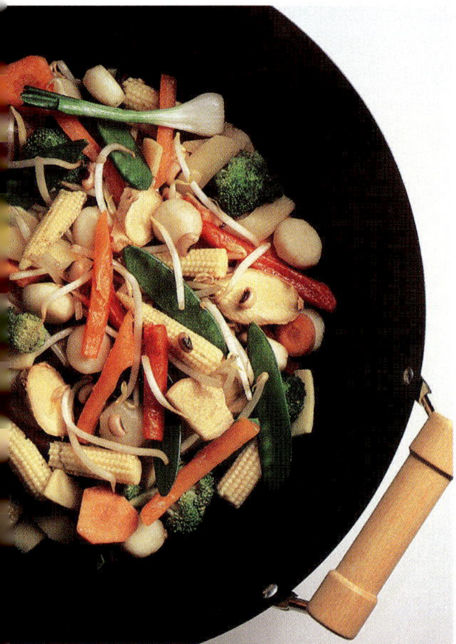

stir-fry vegetables

Mediterranean sardines

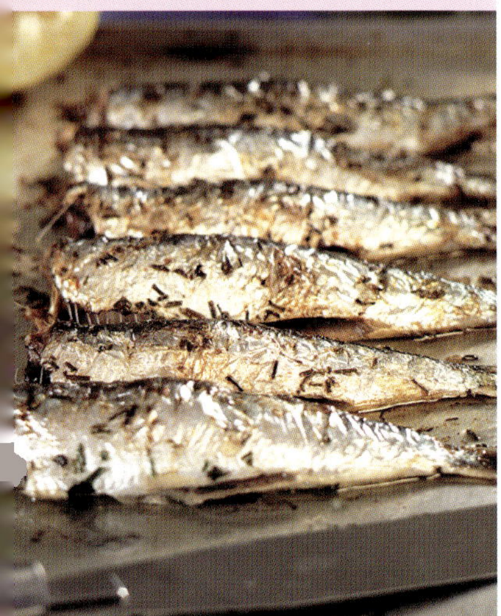

## Watch those fats

- Try not using any spread sometimes, for example with beans on toast.
- For sandwiches too, the bread doesn't need to be buttered if the filling is moist. Alternatively, mustard, chutney or cranberry sauce make good spreads in place of a fat spread.
- Use semi-skimmed or skimmed milk rather than whole (full-fat) milk in drinks, on cereals, in sauces and in milk puddings.
- Thicken sauces with cornflour (blended with a little water) rather than a fat and flour roux.
- Swap cream for low-fat yogurt, creamy tasting reduced-fat Greek-style yogurt or low-fat fromage frais. For stirring into a soup, casserole or curry, blend 1 tbsp yogurt with 1 tsp cornflour to prevent it from curdling.
- Red meat is an excellent source of high quality protein iron, and vitamin $B_{12}$ but choose lean cuts and trim off any visible fat.
- Remove the skin from poultry as this will reduce the fat content significantly.
- Buy yourself a good non-stick pan so you can pan-fry with just a small amount of oil, if needed. Minced meat doesn't require any fat to be added to the pan. Cooking on a hot griddle also requires very little fat – brush the food with a little oil, not the pan.
- Choose low-fat cooking methods, like grilling, baking, poaching, microwaving or stir-frying. Do not deep-fry food or cook in batter.
- Roast or grill meat on a rack so that the fat drips through underneath.
- Put fish on the menu. It needs little preparation and is fast and easy to cook – grill, poach, bake or pan-fry. All fish is low in saturated fat, but oily types like salmon, sardines and mackerel also contain omega-3 fatty acids, which are good for the heart. Eat fish at least twice a week, including one portion of oily fish.
- If a recipe uses hard cheese, use a small amount of a mature-flavoured one, like Parmesan, Stilton or mature Cheddar that will add lots of flavour without needing to use too much.

# Your superhealthy eating plan

Week two

| | BREAKFAST | LUNCH | DINNER |
|---|---|---|---|
| FRIDAY | Bacon and tomato ciabatta. Toasted ciabatta or French bread (unbuttered) filled with lean grilled bacon and thickly sliced grilled tomatoes | Guacamole, tomato salsa or tzatziki dip with a selection of raw vegetable crudités and sesame seed grissini. Wedge of fresh pineapple. | Char-grilled tuna loin with fine green beans and sliced, boiled potatoes. Marinate tuna in a little olive oil, flavoured with chopped fresh chilli and rosemary then grill or cook on a griddle. Raspberries topped with half-fat crème fraiche. |
| SATURDAY | Porridge made with semi-skimmed milk, topped with sliced banana and drizzled with a little honey. | Sardines on toast (see page 31). Blueberry muffin. | Tandoori chicken, chicken tikka kebab or prawn curry with plain or pilau rice, chapatti, cucumber raita and salad. Fresh mango or lychees or sorbet. |
| SUNDAY | Smoked salmon with scrambled egg. Whisk eggs with a little semi-skimmed milk and freshly ground black pepper then cook gently in a non-stick pan with just a small knob of butter or in the microwave, until softly set. Stir in strips of smoked salmon. Serve on wholemeal toast (unbuttered). Glass of tomato juice. | Oatcakes (unbuttered) with camembert or reduced-fat soft cheese. Handful of grapes. | Casserole (made with lean meat or skinned chicken) with rice or boiled new potatoes and selection of seasonal vegetables. Fresh fruit salad topped with reduced-fat Greek-style yogurt or natural bio yogurt. |

### FOR DINNER

- Use less meat in casseroles and bulk up the quantity with extra vegetables.
- Vegetables are great for adding to curries and stir-fries.
- Add extra vegetables, like onions, peppers and mushrooms, to pizza toppings. Pineapple is also good for a fruity choice.
- Add chopped vegetables to a home-made tomato sauce for serving with pasta. You can give it a quick burst in a processor if you need to camouflage the vegetables!
- Some vegetables, such as courgettes, marrow, beef tomatoes, and sweet peppers are perfect for stuffing. Simply scoop out the seeds, fill with a tasty rice or lean minced meat mixture then bake.
- Make fruit or vegetable kebabs to cook on the barbecue.
- Serve a side salad with your meals, but go easy on the dressing.
- Fruits, such as mango, pineapple and kiwi also make delicious fruity salsas, chopped with fresh mint and ginger, for serving with cold cuts and smoked fish.
- Canned fruits in natural juice are useful for instant desserts. For example, try plums or raspberries puréed then swirled together with reduced-fat Greek-style yogurt.

### FOR SNACKS

- Cut up raw carrots, celery or peppers and serve as crudités with a tomato salsa or tzatziki dip.
- Dried fruit, such as ready-to-eat apricots and prunes or jumbo raisins, is ideal for snacking. However dried fruit is high in the natural sugar, fructose, and is therefore quite high in calories so don't choose this option too freely.

## FROZEN V FRESH

Commercially produced frozen foods are frozen immediately after harvesting when the nutrient levels are at their highest so frozen fruit and vegetables are certainly as good, if not better, than fresh. After harvesting, vitamin C levels start to drop as it is sensitive to heat, light and air. It's therefore best to buy fresh produce regularly, keep it in a cool dark place and to eat it soon after purchase.

## CAREFUL COOKING

Vitamin C is the least stable of all the vitamins and easily destroyed during the preparation and cooking of food. It is water-soluble so to preserve the maximum amount of the vitamin, cook fruits and vegetables in only a small amount of water for the minimum time, until just tender. Wherever possible use the cooking water for making gravy, stock or soup. Stewed fruits can be served with their cooking juice. Alternatively, steaming, microwaving and stir-frying are excellent cooking methods for preserving vital nutrients.

## Week three

| | BREAKFAST | LUNCH | DINNER |
|---|---|---|---|
| MONDAY | Fresh grapefruit or grapefruit segments (unsweetened). Sugar-free muesli or wholegrain cereal with semi-skimmed milk | Greek salad. Make with chopped cucumber, tomatoes, peppers, red onions, feta cheese, olives and rocket sprinkled with a little olive oil, lemon juice, oregano and freshly ground black pepper. | Spaghetti bolognese. Make bolognese sauce using lean beef or turkey mince with chopped onions, carrots, celery, peppers, tomatoes and peas. Serve with wholewheat spaghetti and sprinkle with a little freshly grated Parmesan. |
| TUESDAY | Prunes (or dried fruit compote) with reduced-fat Greek-style yogurt. Soak dried fruit in Earl Grey tea or apple juice or use canned prunes in fruit juice. If liked, add some orange and grapefruit segments. | Falafel pitta. Falafel, chickpea croquettes, are sold in Middle Eastern cafés and delis or can be bought chilled from the supermarket. Serve hot in warm pitta spread with harissa (chilli sauce) with salad and hummus (see page 23). Slice of watermelon or other fresh fruit. | Grilled beefburger, made with lean minced beef. Serve with beetroot and onion relish, watercress salad and potato wedges. |
| WEDNESDAY | Tomatoes on toast. Use drained, canned plum tomatoes or thickly sliced fresh tomatoes on wholemeal toast. | Roast chicken salad. Toss skinned and sliced roast chicken breast with mixed salad leaves, lightly cooked asparagus tips, sliced peaches or nectarines and a little French dressing. | Tagliatelle with prawns. Start with a tomato sauce for pasta then add chopped mushrooms, peppers, olives, sun-dried tomatoes and prawns. Flavour with garlic, fresh herbs or chilli. |

## How to do it

Including more fruit and vegetables in your diet couldn't be easier. There's no need to make major changes to your lifestyle – simply add them to your meals and use them for snacks, if you're feeling peckish during the day. For maximum benefit, eat a wide variety. With so many delicious choices throughout the seasons, there's always something for all tastes. Many people think they're not keen on vegetables, probably as a result of eating over-cooked, unappetising ones some time in the past. If so, take a fresh look at quick cooking methods and exciting new serving suggestions, and you'll soon be converted. Here are some ideas to get you started.

### FOR BREAKFAST

- Mash a small banana and spread it on wholemeal toast.
- Make a delicious smoothie by blending sliced banana, strawberries, raspberries, peach or mango with semi-skimmed milk and low-fat yogurt.
- For a non-dairy smoothie, simply blend a selection of soft fruits without the milk and yogurt.
- Scatter blueberries, strawberries, raspberries or sliced banana or peaches over a bowl of cereal or porridge.
- Serve grilled tomatoes or baked beans on wholemeal toast.
- Juice your own fresh fruits.

### FOR LUNCH

- Make a pasta salad and add chopped peppers, sweetcorn and tomatoes.
- Pack out sandwiches with plenty of salad.
- Vegetables make a great-tasting soup and are frequently sold in take-away bars. For home-made, simply sauté chopped vegetables (such as onions, leeks, carrots, tomatoes, swede, celeriac, parsnip, sprouts or broccoli) in a pan with a little oil / butter then add stock, flavour with herbs or spices and cook until tender. Serve chunky or process for a smooth soup. Pack in a thermos flask.
- Finish off your lunch with a piece of fresh fruit, a fruit salad or some fruit stirred into reduced-fat Greek-style yogurt.

**Eating at least 5 portions of fruit and vegetables a day is a positive way to be healthier, as it concentrates on what you can eat rather than what you should cut out from your diet. As the vast majority of fruit and vegetables contain no fat and are also very low in calories, they're the ultimate healthy food if you're trying to lose weight.**

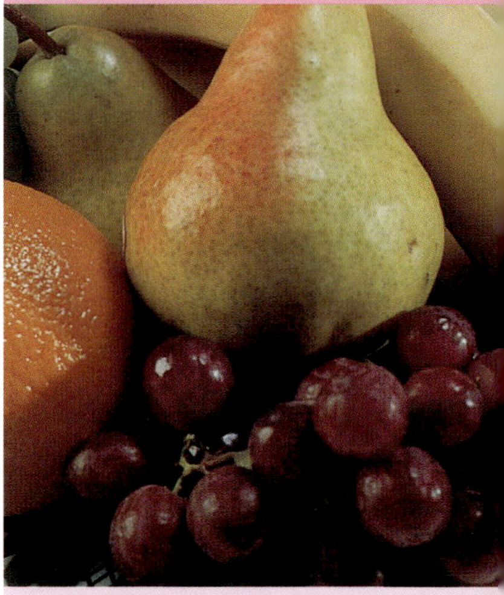

**Choose fruit and vegetables in season for the best value and optimum flavour. Local markets are a good place to shop for the most competitive prices.**

Week three

| | BREAKFAST | LUNCH | DINNER |
|---|---|---|---|
| THURSDAY | Wholegrain cereal or porridge made with semi-skimmed milk. Glass of unsweetened fruit juice. | Tuna and sweetcorn roll. Choose a large wholemeal or multigrain roll and fill with drained and flaked canned tuna mixed with sweetcorn and a little reduced-fat mayonnaise. Add sliced cucumber and rocket leaves. Cherry tomatoes or handful of grapes. | Mixed vegetable curry with brown rice, naan bread or chapatti. |
| FRIDAY | Bagel spread with reduced-fat soft cheese and topped with smoked salmon. Glass of freshly squeezed orange juice. | Sushi selection - available from sushi bars and chilled supermarket cabinets. | Chicken fajitas. Stir-fry strips of seasoned chicken breast with sliced mixed peppers and mushrooms then roll up in warmed tortillas with tomato salsa and a little soured cream. |
| SATURDAY | Half melon filled with mixed red berries (such as fresh strawberries, raspberries and blackcurrants or thawed, frozen fruits of the forest). | Slice of Margherita pizza (thin crust) with Mixed herb salad with toasted nuts and seeds (see page 29). | Garden paella (see page 39). If liked add prawns, mixed shellfish, or chicken breast. |
| SUNDAY | Tropical fruit salad made with papaya, mango, orange and kiwi fruit sprinkled with unsweetened tropical or orange juice. Plus a toasted muffin (unbuttered) topped with peanut butter. | Chicken with roasted vegetables. Cook skinned chicken breasts on a bed of chunky vegetables (such as courgettes, aubergines, onions, peppers and tomatoes). Scatter with thinly sliced garlic and chopped fresh herbs and drizzle with a little olive oil. Baked oaty apples (see page 41). | Herb omelette with grilled tomatoes. Whisk 2 eggs in a bowl with 1 tbsp water, chopped fresh herbs (such as parsley, chives or tarragon) and seasoning. Cook in a non-stick pan with a knob of butter. |

## Why are fruit and vegetables so important?

Eating at least 5 portions of fruit and vegetables a day can help to significantly lower your risk from various diseases such as heart disease, stroke and some cancers. They supply a good mix of nutrients including vitamins A (as beta-carotene), C and E, which act as antioxidants, and fibre, which aids the digestive system. Lightly cooked green vegetables as well as oranges and orange juice also provide a useful source of folic acid. The World Health Organisation (WHO) recommends 400 g (14 oz) of fruit and vegetables a day, which is equal to 5 portions.

## What counts as a portion?

At least 5 portions of fruit and vegetables a day are recommended, with one portion being approximately 80g. Your choices can be fresh, frozen, canned, dried or juiced, although only one glass of juice counts daily.

Potatoes, yam and cassava don't count towards your 5 a day because they are grouped nutritionally with starchy carbohydrates. One portion could be:-

**FRUITS**

- 1 apple, banana, pear, peach or orange
- 1/2 fresh or 3 heaped tbsp canned grapefruit
- 2 plums, fresh apricots or satsumas
- 7 strawberries
- 2 handfuls raspberries or blueberries
- 2 kiwi fruit
- 12 –15 cherries or grapes
- 1 slice melon
- 1 tbsp raisins / sultanas
- 3 ready-to eat dried apricots
- 6 canned prunes
- 2 tbsp stewed or canned fruit (preferably in juice not syrup)
- 3 heaped tbsp fruit salad
- 150 ml glass of fruit (or vegetable) juice or fruit smoothie

**VEGETABLES**

- 3 heaped tbsp cooked carrots, shredded cabbage, peas or sweetcorn
- 3 heaped tbsp beans, chickpeas or lentils
- 5 spears asparagus
- 2 spears broccoli
- 8 Brussels sprouts
- 1 onion or leek
- 3 sticks celery
- 3 handfuls sliced mushrooms
- 2 handfuls bean sprouts
- 1 handful mange-tout
- 1 medium-sized tomato
- 7 cherry tomatoes
- 1/2 sweet pepper
- 1/2 avocado
- 1 cereal bowl of mixed salad

## Hummus

Chickpeas are highly nutritious and very versatile. Blended to make a smooth, creamy dip is a popular way of enjoying them.

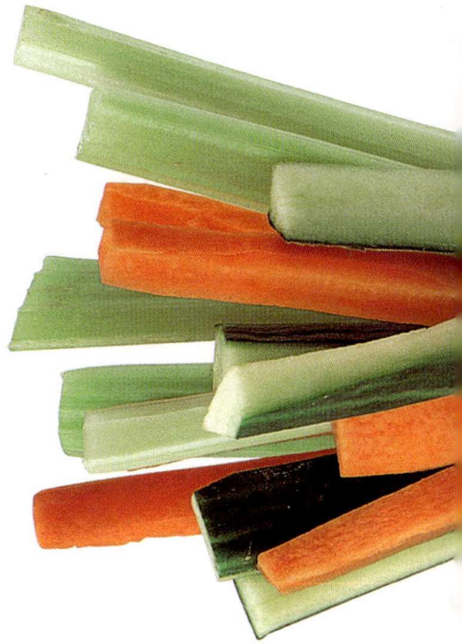

### INGREDIENTS

400 g (14 oz) canned chickpeas, drained and rinsed

2 garlic cloves

2-3 tbsp water

2 tbsp tahini

1 tbsp olive oil

1 lemon, juice

freshly ground black pepper

paprika, to garnish

### DIRECTIONS

1. Place the chickpeas, garlic, water, tahini, olive oil and lemon juice in a food processor. Process until smooth, adding more water or lemon juice if necessary. Season with black pepper.

2. Transfer into a bowl, cover and refrigerate.

3. To serve, garnish with a sprinkling of paprika.

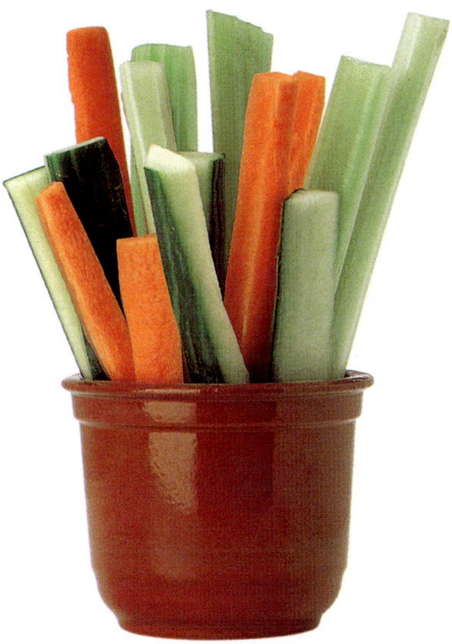

## Crudités

Most vegetables can be eaten raw, and improve the fibre content of a meal when served with a dip such as hummus. Choose a few of the following:

carrot sticks
broccoli or cauliflower florets
celery sticks
cucumber sticks
salad onions
courgette sticks
mange-tout
strips of red, green or yellow pepper
radishes
cherry tomatoes
baby sweetcorn

### RECIPE TIP

Tahini is a paste made from roasted sesame seeds. It has a strong nutty taste. You'll find it in larger supermarkets, delis or continental grocers.

# Snacks & treats

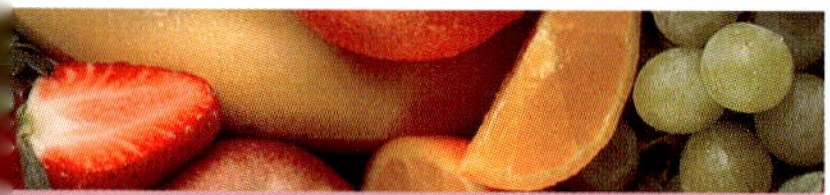

## TEN HEALTHY SNACKS

- Vegetable crudités with tomato salsa or tzatziki dip.
- Piece of fresh fruit or portion of fresh fruit salad (in unsweetened fruit juice).
- 3-4 grissini (breadsticks).
- 2 water biscuits or oatcakes thinly spread with yeast extract or low-fat soft cheese.
- Handful of cherry tomatoes with 6 stoned olives.
- 5 Brazil nuts, dates or ready-to-eat dried apricots.
- Virgin Mary – tomato juice with Tabasco and Worcestershire sauce served with a stick of celery.
- Mug of vegetable (non-creamy) soup.
- 125 g pot of low-fat or natural bio yogurt
- Fruit ice lolly made with unsweetened fruit juice.

One of the biggest problems when following a diet is learning to change your eating habits. Whereas you may be used to grabbing a bar of chocolate or a bag of crisps between meals or raiding the biscuit tin while slumped in front of the TV in the evening, you now have to be prepared to make healthy choices. The main thing to remember is not to skip meals so you're less likely to be hungry between meals. However if you do find you are peckish at any time, that's not a problem. Rather than buying cakes, biscuits, crisps and sweets, shop for healthy snacks so you always have something satisfying ready to hand for weak moments.

## TREATS

You can occasionally indulge yourself with one of these tempting treats, but remember, they add unnecessary calories to your diet. Cut out such foods and drinks to lose weight faster or step up your exercise routine to help burn more calories.

- 1 standard glass (125 ml) of wine.
- half a pint lager / cider / beer / shandy.
- 1 spirit measure (25 ml) with diet mixer.
- 1 standard packet of crisps.
- 2 digestive biscuits.
- Slice of malt loaf, a toasted wholemeal hot cross bun with a lick of butter or a small piece of fruity flapjack.
- 1 fun-size chocolate bar.
- Small portion of dairy ice-cream.
- Fruit crudités (chunks of fresh fruit) with chocolate dip (melt just a couple of squares of dark chocolate and stir into reduced-fat Greek-style yogurt).

## Tomato & Courgette Soup

Tomatoes form the base of many vegetable soups. As well as being a good source of vitamin C, they contain the powerful antioxidant, lycopene. Use full-flavoured tomatoes, preferably vine-ripened, for the best flavour.

**SERVES 2 as a light lunch or**
**SERVES 4 as a starter**

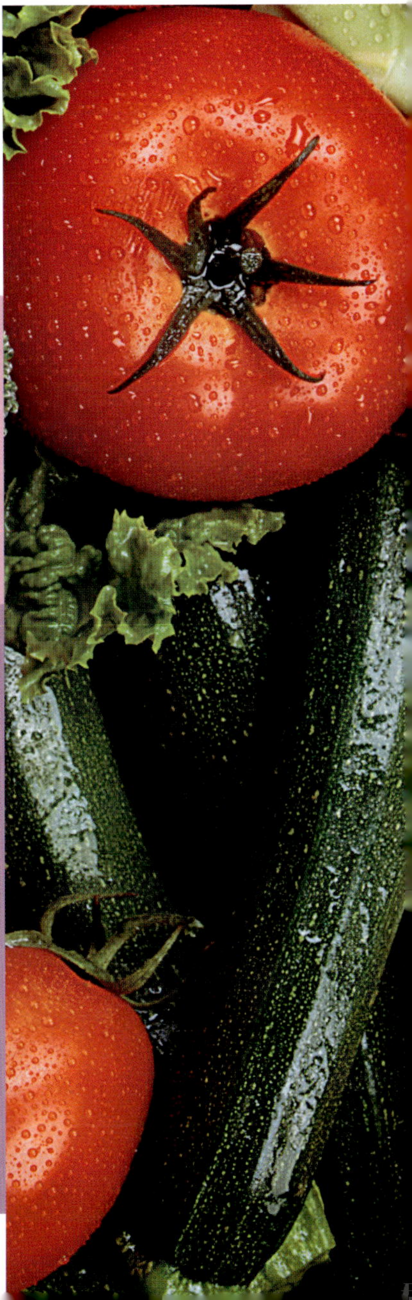

### INGREDIENTS

- 450 g (1 lb) ripe tomatoes
- 1 litre (1¾ pints) vegetable stock
- 1 onion, finely chopped
- 2 garlic cloves, finely chopped
- freshly ground black pepper
- 225 g (8 oz) courgettes
- 1 tsp olive oil
- handful fresh basil leaves, roughly chopped

### DIRECTIONS

1. Using a sharp knife, make crosses in the tops of the tomatoes and put them into a heatproof bowl. Pour over boiling water and leave for 2 minutes. Drain the tomatoes, then skin them, chop finely and leave to one side.

2. Heat a little of the vegetable stock in a heavy saucepan and gently cook the onion and garlic until translucent. Add the chopped tomatoes and rest of the stock. Bring to the boil, cover and simmer gently for 20 minutes. Season to taste with pepper. Cut the courgettes into small cubes, add to the soup and bring to boiling point. Allow to bubble for 2 minutes until the courgettes are just tender. Drizzle in the olive oil.

3. To serve, ladle into a bowl and sprinkle the basil leaves on top.

## Baked Oaty Apples

A fabulous fruity recipe that shows how by making healthy choices, you can even enjoy delicious puddings on a diet.

SERVES 2

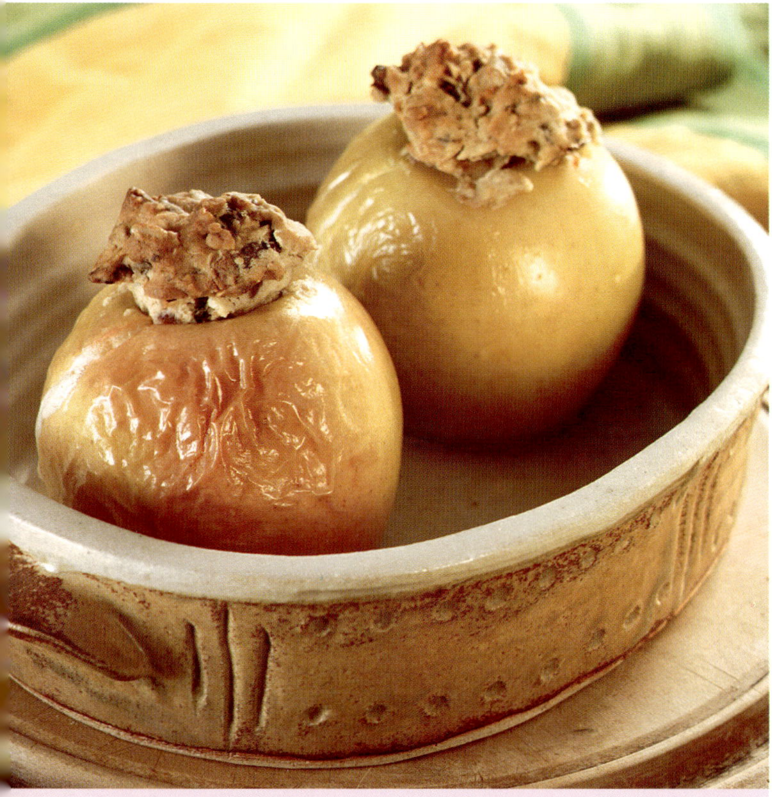

### INGREDIENTS

40 g (1½ oz) flour

2 tbsp unsalted butter

2 tbsp porridge oats

2 tbsp runny honey

1 tbsp sunflower seeds

50 g (2 oz) dates, finely chopped

2 large baking apples, cored

100 ml (3½ fl oz) unsweetened apple juice

### DIRECTIONS

1. Preheat the oven to 180°C/350°F/Gas Mark 4. Mix together the flour, butter, oats, honey, sunflower seeds and dates in a bowl. Fill the cavity of each apple with the oat mixture.

2. Place the apples in an oven-proof dish and pour the apple juice around. Bake for 45 minutes or until the apples are tender, basting with the juice from time to time.

### RECIPE TIPS

You can ring the changes with the stuffing mixture by adding chopped ready-to-eat dried apricots, sultanas or mincemeat in place of the dates. A pinch of ground cinnamon could be added for a spicy flavour.

## Grilled Vegetable Soup

This combination of smoky aubergines, red peppers, tomatoes, garlic and herbs makes the quintessential Mediterranean soup, which is packed with vitamins. Add grilled courgettes for variety.

### SERVES 4

### DIRECTIONS

1. Place the onion, garlic, tomatoes, aubergines and peppers under a preheated hot grill for about 10 minutes until charred and softened. Leave to cool slightly, then peel the onion, garlic and tomatoes. Remove any charred skin from the aubergines and peppers. Roughly chop the flesh.

2. Gently heat the olive oil with the thyme and bay leaf in a large, heavy-based saucepan for 2 minutes. Add the chopped vegetables, sun-dried tomatoes and stock. Bring to the boil, cover and simmer gently for 20 minutes.

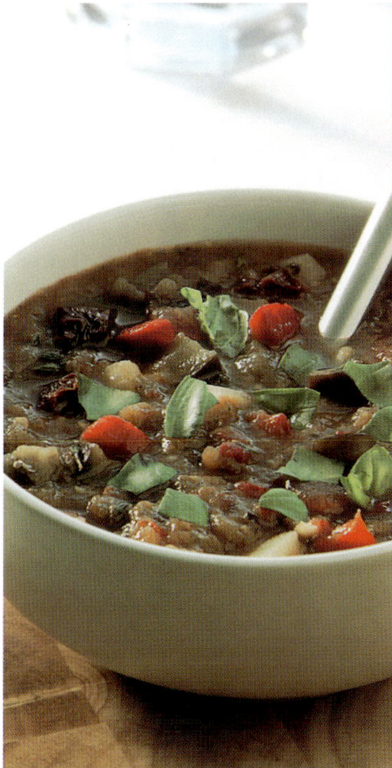

### INGREDIENTS

1 onion, halved but not peeled

4 garlic cloves

4 ripe tomatoes

2 aubergines, halved lengthways

2 red peppers, halved and deseeded

1 tbsp olive oil

5 sprigs fresh thyme

1 bay leaf

4 sun-dried tomatoes, chopped

1 litre ($1^{3}/_{4}$ pints) vegetable stock

$^{1}/_{2}$ lemon, freshly squeezed

freshly ground black pepper

handful fresh basil leaves, torn

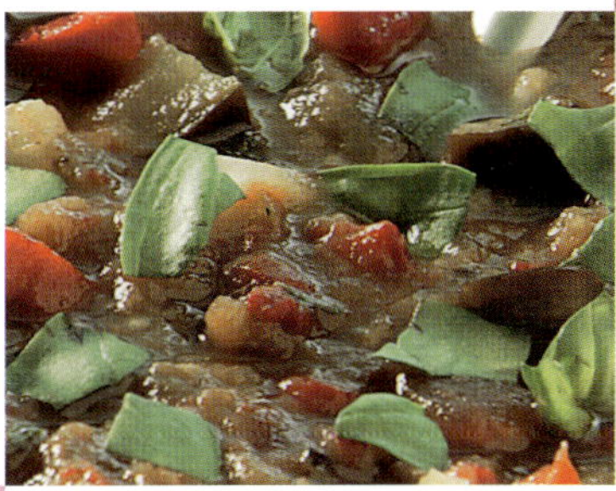

3. Leave to cool then remove the herbs. Transfer the soup into a food processor and process briefly to retain some of the vegetables' texture.

4. Return the soup to the pan, squeeze in the lemon juice and season to taste with pepper and reheat.

5. To serve, garnish with torn basil leaves.

## Raspberry & Oat Crunch

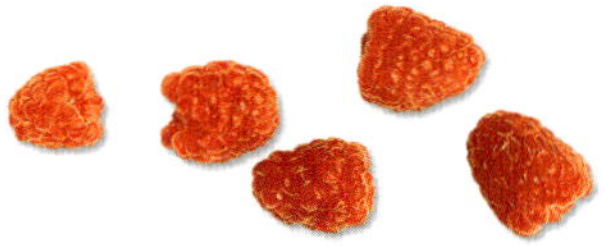

This pudding looks stunning but is very simple to make. It also makes a nutritious breakfast containing calcium, and vitamins B and C.

SERVES 2

### INGREDIENTS

40 g (1½ oz) porridge oats

1 tbsp sunflower seeds

250 g (9 oz) thick natural bio yogurt or reduced-fat Greek-style yogurt

1 tbsp honey or maple syrup

115 g (4 oz) fresh or frozen raspberries (defrost before using)

### DIRECTIONS

1. Place the porridge oats and sunflower seeds in a large, heavy-based frying pan and roast over a medium heat for 1–2 minutes until lightly toasted. Leave to cool.

2. Place the yogurt in a large bowl and stir in the honey or maple syrup. Add the raspberries and fold in gently.

3. Stir in the oats and sunflower seeds, leaving a few to sprinkle on top. Spoon the mixture into 2 glasses and sprinkle with the reserved oats and seeds before serving.

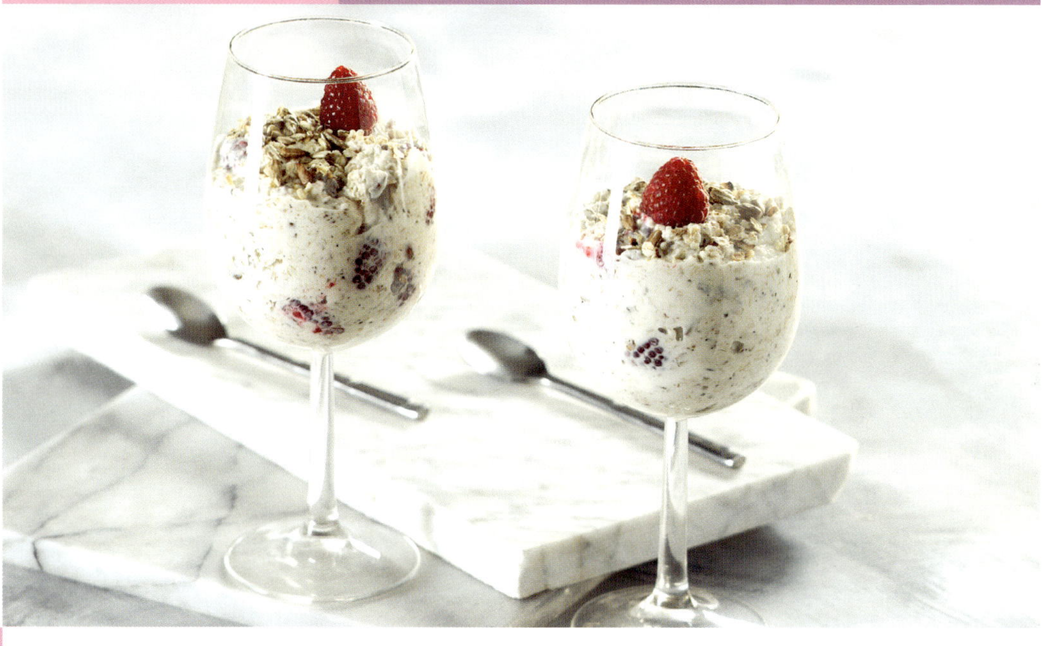

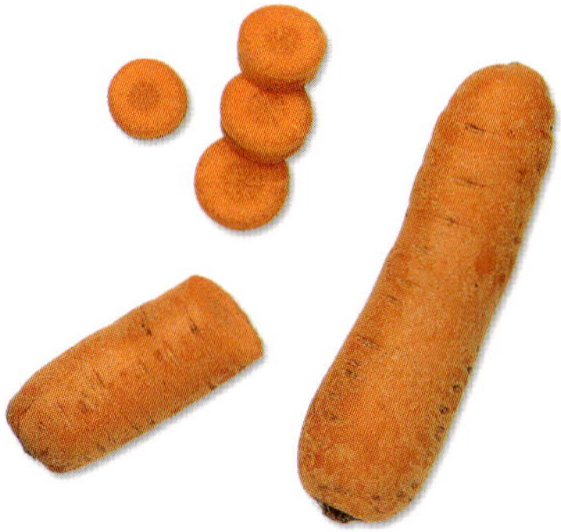

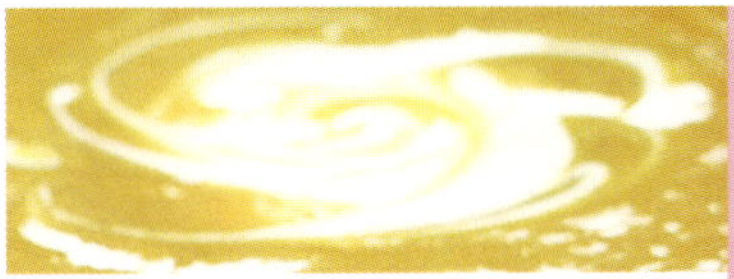

## Lentil & Carrot Soup

This nutritious soup makes a filling and wholesome lunch or supper, served with good wholemeal, mixed grain or soda bread.

SERVES 2

### INGREDIENTS

1 tbsp olive oil

1 onion, chopped

2 garlic cloves, chopped

1 tsp each ground cumin, ginger and turmeric

2 carrots, sliced

115 g (4 oz) red lentils

600 ml (1 pint) vegetable stock

salt and freshly ground pepper

2 tbsp live natural bio yogurt, to serve

### DIRECTIONS

1. Heat the oil in a saucepan, add the onion and lightly sauté for 8-10 minutes until softened. Add the garlic and spices and cook for 1 minute.

2. Add the carrots and lentils and cook for 2 minutes, stirring continuously.

3. Pour in the stock and bring to the boil. Reduce the heat and simmer for 40 minutes. Blend or process until smooth and creamy, adding more stock or water if required. Season to taste and serve with a spoonful of yogurt on top.

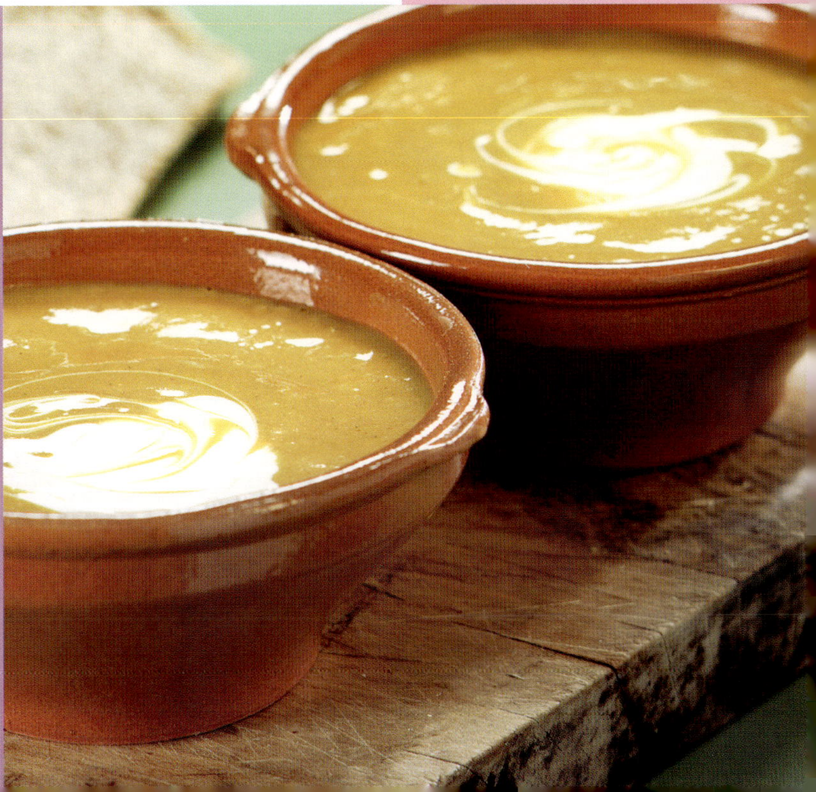

## Garden Paella

A twist on the classic Spanish dish. If liked, add some prawns, mixed shellfish or cooked pieces of chicken.

SERVES 4

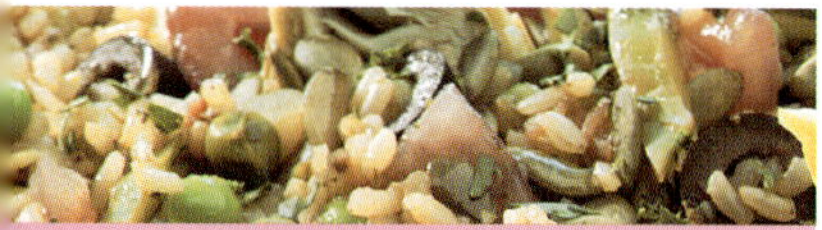

### INGREDIENTS

600 ml (1 pint) vegetable stock

1 onion, finely chopped

2 garlic cloves, crushed

200 g (8 oz) long-grain brown rice

115g (4 oz) peas (fresh or frozen)

115 g (4 oz) green beans, sliced

400 g (14 oz) can artichoke hearts, drained and halved

6 strands saffron

6 tomatoes, skinned and chopped

1 tsp dried oregano

1 tbsp chopped fresh thyme

2 tbsp finely chopped fresh parsley, plus extra to garnish

black pepper

1 lemon, juice

12 black or green olives, halved

2 tbsp pumpkin seeds

lemon wedges, to garnish

### DIRECTIONS

1. Heat a little of the stock in a large saucepan and sauté the onion and garlic until soft.

2. Add the rice and cook gently for 1 minute. Add the peas, beans and artichoke hearts, stirring well, and cook over a very low heat for 4–5 minutes.

3. Bring the rest of the stock to the boil in another pan, dissolve the saffron in the boiling stock, then add to the pan with the tomatoes and herbs.

4. Bring to the boil, reduce the heat and cook, uncovered, for about 30 minutes, stirring frequently. Add more liquid if necessary, stirring frequently, until the rice is tender. Add more liquid if necessary.

5. Season with black pepper and add the lemon juice. Stir in the olives and pumpkin seeds, garnish with chopped parsley and lemon wedges, and serve hot.

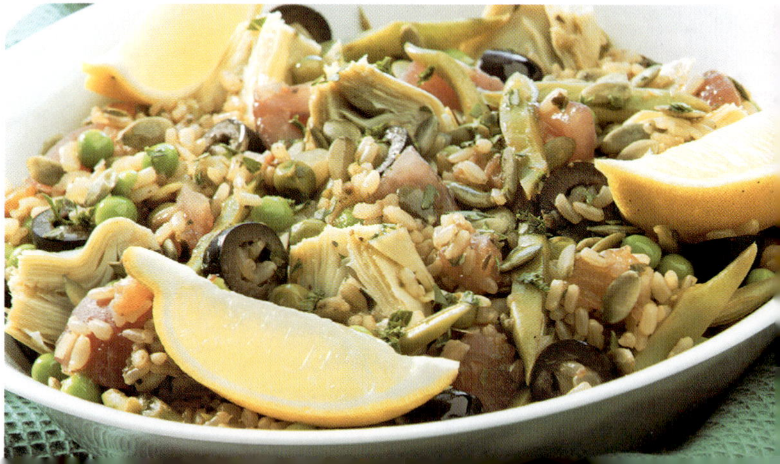

## Chickpea & Tomato Salad

Chickpeas are high in vegetable protein. Add some cubes of feta, grilled smoked tofu or goat's cheese for a complete meal.

SERVES 4

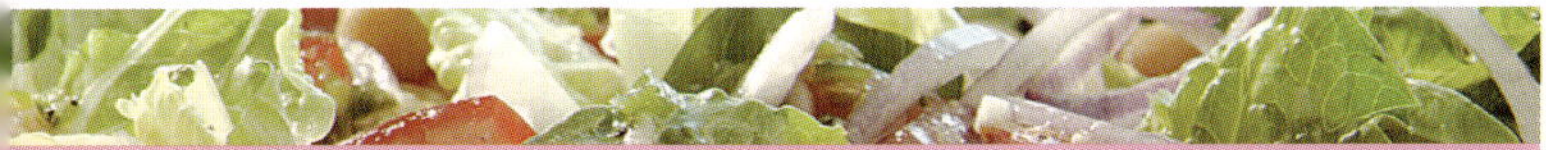

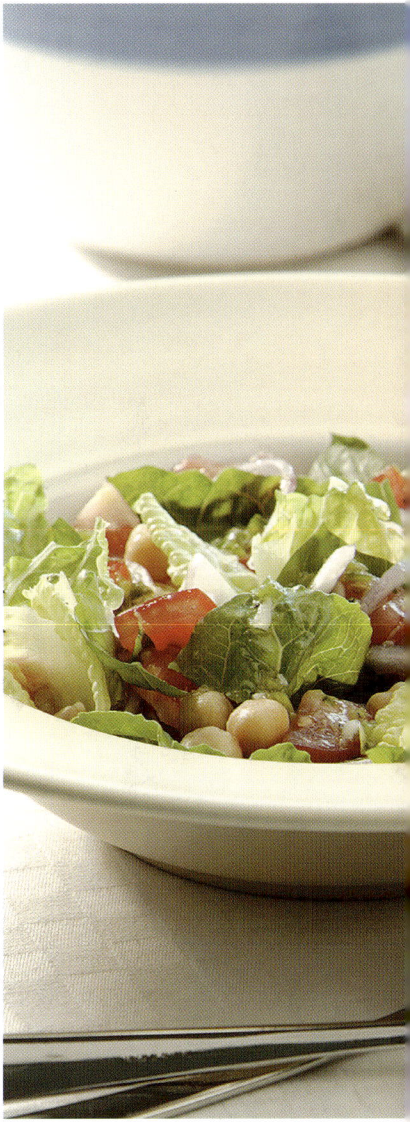

### INGREDIENTS

- 175 g (6 oz) dried chickpeas or 400 g (14 oz) canned, drained and rinsed
- 1 green chilli, deseeded and finely chopped
- 1 garlic clove, crushed
- 2 lemons, juice and zest
- 2 tbsp olive oil
- 1 tbsp water
- freshly ground black pepper
- 225 g (8 oz) ripe tomatoes, roughly chopped
- 1 red onion, thinly sliced
- handful fresh basil leaves, torn
- 1 cos or romaine lettuce, torn

### DIRECTIONS

1. If using dried chickpeas, soak overnight then boil for at least 30 minutes until soft. Leave to cool.

2. Put the chilli, garlic, lemon zest and juice, olive oil, water and black pepper in a screwtop-jar and shake vigorously. Taste and add more lemon juice or oil if necessary.

3.Add the tomatoes, onion and basil to the chickpeas and mix gently. Pour over the dressing and mix again. To serve, arrange on a bed of lettuce.

## Stuffed Vegetables

A delicious vegetarian recipe that will boost your 5 a day intake. Choose your favourite vegetables to stuff.

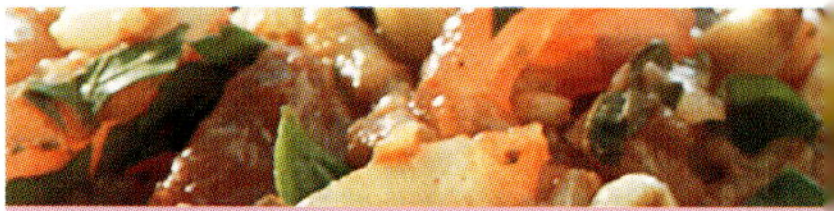

**INGREDIENTS**

2 peppers, 2 medium aubergines, 2 large courgettes or 4 beef tomatoes

1 tbsp vegetable oil

1 small onion, chopped

2 garlic cloves, crushed

1 tbsp tomato purée

6 ripe tomatoes, skinned and chopped

4 tbsp cooked brown rice

25 g (1 oz) pine nuts, lightly toasted

1 tbsp chopped fresh parsley

1 tbsp chopped fresh mint

1 tbsp chopped fresh basil

1/4 tsp ground cinnamon

1 lemon, juice

freshly ground black pepper

**SERVES 2**

**DIRECTIONS**

1. Preheat the oven to 180°C/350°F/Gas Mark 4.

• If stuffing aubergines or courgettes, trim the stems, then halve lengthways. Use a teaspoon to hollow out each half, leaving a shell about 1 cm (1/2 in) thick. Chop the scooped-out flesh. Steam the shells over boiling water for about 4 minutes, then hold under cold water to stop further cooking and dry with kitchen paper.

• If stuffing peppers, slice off the tops (put to one side) and scoop out and discard the seeds.

• If stuffing tomatoes, slice off the tops (put to one side) and scoop out the seeds and flesh, and add the latter to the rice mixture in step 2.

2. Heat the oil in a non-stick frying pan, add the onions and garlic and sauté, stirring, until translucent. Stir in the tomato purée, tomatoes, chopped aubergine or courgette flesh (if using), cooked rice, pine nuts, herbs and cinnamon and continue cooking for a couple of minutes.

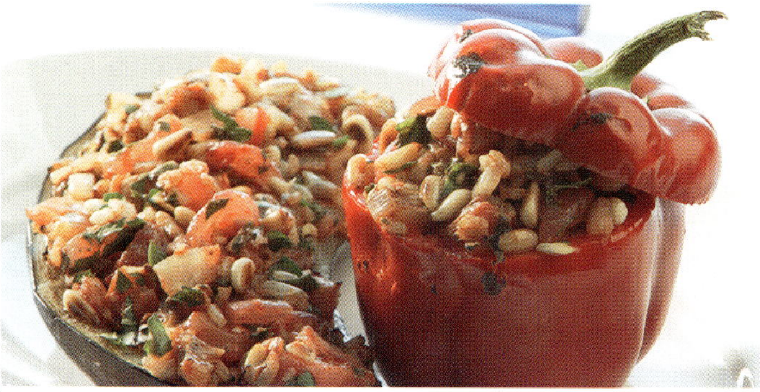

3. Stir in the lemon juice and season to taste with pepper.

4. Stuff the vegetables with the rice mixture and put the lids back on the peppers or tomatoes. Place in a lightly greased baking dish and bake for about 20 minutes.

## Watercress, Orange & Walnut Salad

A colourful and, refreshing side salad, providing iron, beta-carotene and vitamins C and E.

SERVES 2

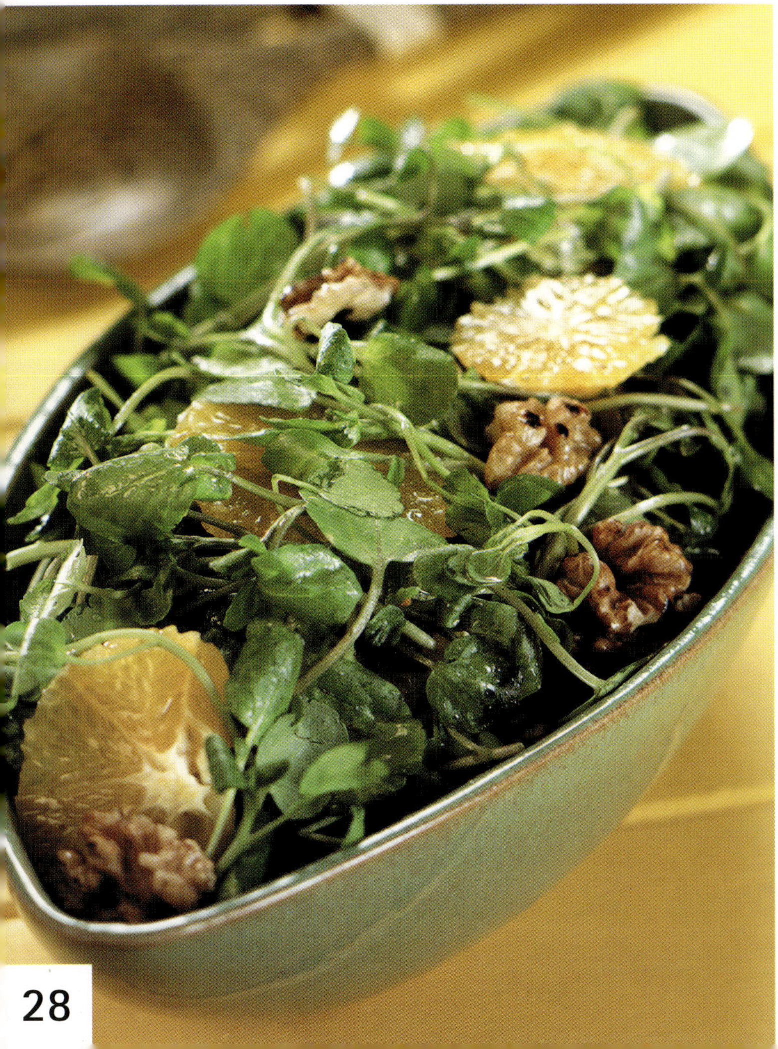

### INGREDIENTS

50 g (2 oz) shelled walnuts, halved

75 g (3 oz) watercress, tough stalks removed

1 large orange, peeled and sliced into thin rounds

### DRESSING

2 tsp lemon juice

$^{1}/_{2}$ tsp runny honey

1 tsp Dijon mustard

1$^{1}/_{2}$ tbsp extra virgin olive oil

salt and freshly ground pepper

### DIRECTIONS

1. Lightly toast the walnuts in a dry frying pan for 2 minutes until slightly golden. Toss them frequently to prevent burning. Leave to cool.

2. To make the dressing, whisk the lemon juice, honey and mustard together in a bowl. Gradually whisk in the olive oil and season to taste with salt and pepper.

3. Place the watercress, orange slices and walnuts in a salad bowl. Pour the dressing over and toss well.

## Spanish Omelette

A delicious lunch or supper dish. Serve hot or cold with a salad.

SERVES 2

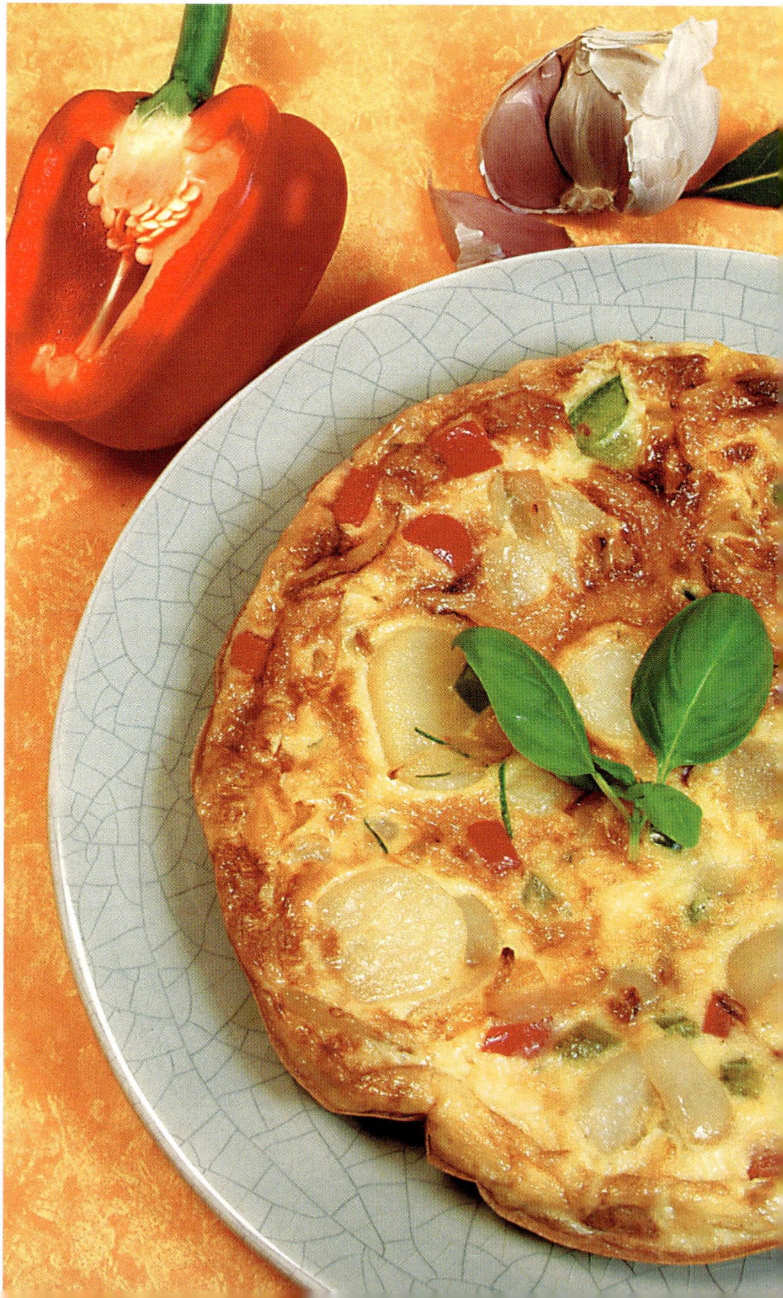

### INGREDIENTS

1 tbsp olive oil

1 onion, sliced

1 garlic clove, crushed

½ pepper deseeded and chopped

450g (1 lb) new potatoes, cooked and diced

4 eggs, beaten

freshly ground black pepper

### DIRECTIONS

1. Heat the oil in a non-stick frying pan and gently sauté the onion, garlic and peppers for 4-5 minutes.

2. Add the potatoes and continue to sauté until golden.

3. Season the eggs then pour over the vegetables and cook gently until set. Finish off under a preheated grill.

## Mixed Herb Salad with Toasted Nuts & Seeds

No need for green salads to be dull. Add fresh herbs, toasted nuts and seeds for an exciting combination.

SERVES 2

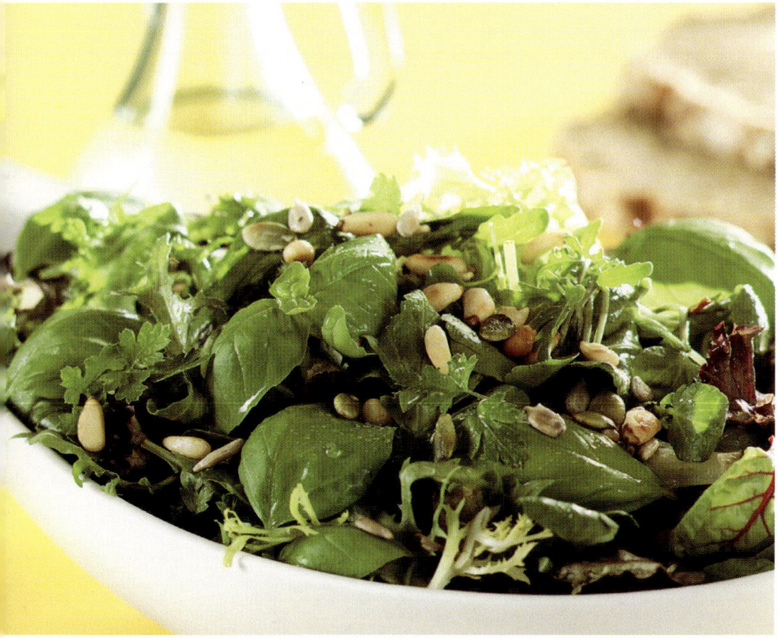

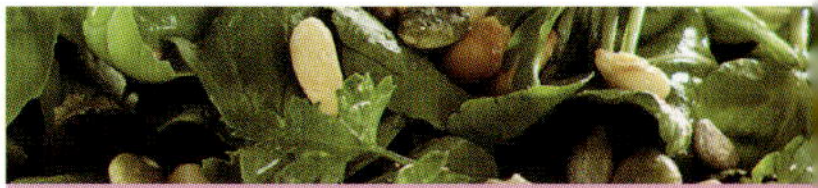

### INGREDIENTS

50 g (2 oz) mixed salad leaves, including watercress and baby spinach

50 g (2 oz) mixed herbs, including parsley, rocket and basil

1 tbsp sunflower seeds

1 tbsp pumpkin seeds

1 tbsp pine nuts

### DRESSING

2 tbsp extra virgin olive oil

1–2 tsp fresh lemon juice

salt and freshly ground pepper

### DIRECTIONS

1. Arrange the salad leaves and herbs in a serving bowl. Lightly toast the seeds and pine nuts in a dry frying pan until just coloured. Leave them to cool slightly before sprinkling over the salad.

2. Mix together the olive oil and lemon juice. Season to taste with salt and pepper and drizzle over the salad.

### HEALTH TIP

A salad is an easy and tasty way of helping you to reach your 5 a day target of fruit and vegetables.

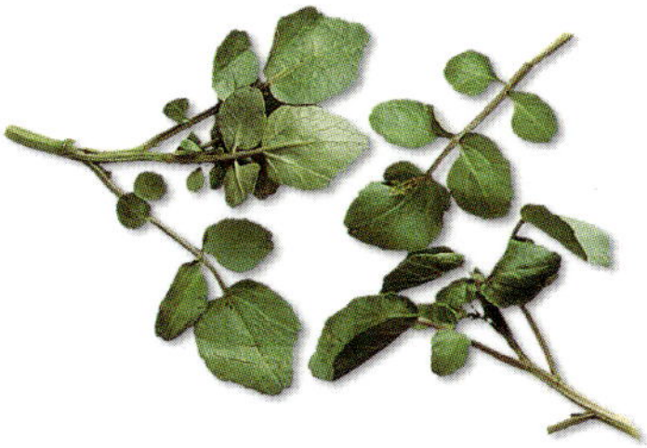

## Penne with Char-Grilled Peppers, Broccoli & Pine Nuts

This nutritious recipe contains plenty of antioxidant vitamins, is quick to prepare and very satisfying to eat. Ideal for an easy mid-week meal.

**SERVES 4**

### INGREDIENTS

1 red and 1 yellow pepper, deseeded and quartered

350 g (12 oz) wholewheat penne pasta

1 head broccoli, divided into small florets

½ onion, finely chopped

2 garlic cloves, crushed

1 tbsp vegetable oil

1 tbsp tomato purée

25 g (1 oz) pine nuts

12 black olives, stoned and sliced

1 tbsp shredded fresh basil, plus extra to garnish

freshly ground black pepper

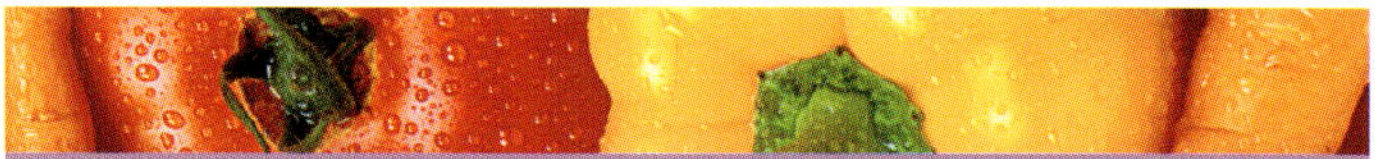

### DIRECTIONS

1. Place the peppers under a hot grill and grill, skin-side up, until the skin begins to char. Place in a plastic bag, leave to cool then remove the skin and cut the flesh into strips.

2. Fill a large saucepan with water, add a pinch of salt and bring to the boil. Cook the pasta for 10-12 minutes or according to the instructions on the packet until tender, then drain.

3. Steam the broccoli for 5 minutes until just tender.

4. Sauté the onions and garlic in the oil for about 5 minutes or until the onion is translucent. Stir in the peppers then mix in the tomato purée. Add the broccoli, pine nuts, olives and basil, and season with black pepper. Heat gently for 2 minutes, then stir in the pasta.

5. Transfer to a serving dish and garnish with torn basil leaves.

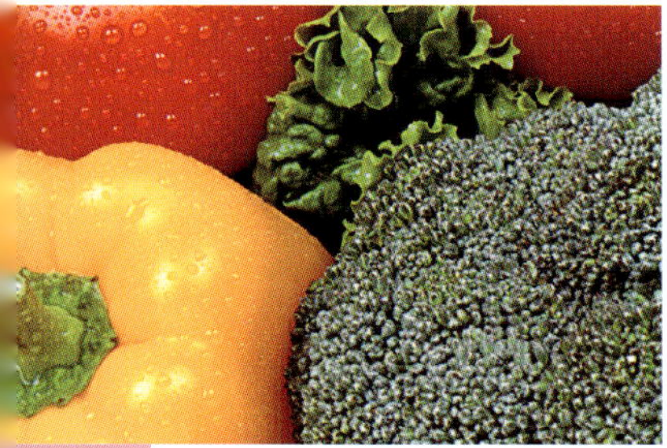

### RECIPE TIP

Putting the char-grilled peppers into a plastic bag while hot, creates steam and loosens the skins so they are easy to remove.

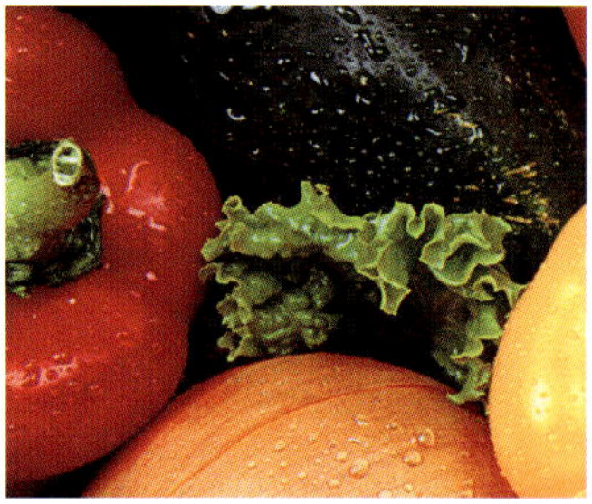

## Sweetcorn & Tomato Salsa

A satisfying variation on the more usual tomato salsa that makes an appealing side dish.

SERVES 2

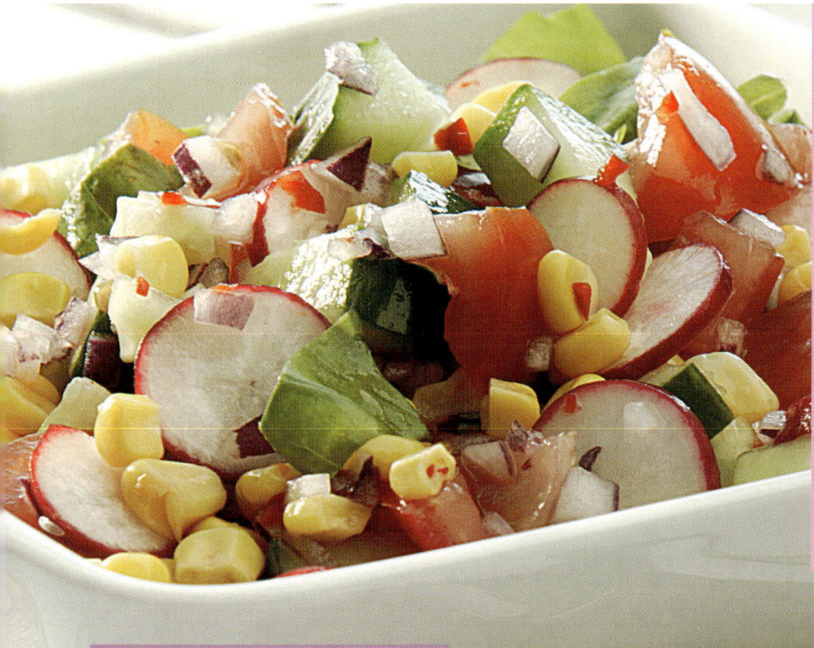

### INGREDIENTS

115 g (4 oz) frozen sweetcorn

1/2 red onion, finely chopped

1/2 red chilli, deseeded and finely chopped

115 g (4 oz) ripe tomatoes, chopped

1/2 cucumber, chopped

4 radishes, sliced

1 tbsp fresh basil, roughly shredded

1 lime, juice

freshly ground black pepper

### DIRECTIONS

1. Defrost and cook the sweetcorn according to the packet instructions and leave to cool.

2. Mix all the ingredients together, cover and leave to stand at room temperature for at least an hour before serving.

## Chilli con Carne

A great family favourite and also an ideal dish for easy entertaining. Serve with brown or basmati rice, jacket potatoes or reduced-fat garlic bread and a crisp salad or Sweetcorn & tomato salsa (see page 30).

**SERVES 4**

### INGREDIENTS

- 450g (1 lb) lean minced beef
- 1 large onion, chopped
- 2 garlic cloves, crushed
- 1 red pepper, deseeded and chopped
- 400g (14 oz) can chopped tomatoes
- 1 tbsp tomato purée
- 1 bay leaf
- 1 tsp ground cumin
- $\frac{1}{2}$ tsp chilli powder (or to taste)
- 1 tsp yeast extract
- 150ml (5 fl oz) beef stock
- 425g (15 oz) can red kidney beans, drained and rinsed

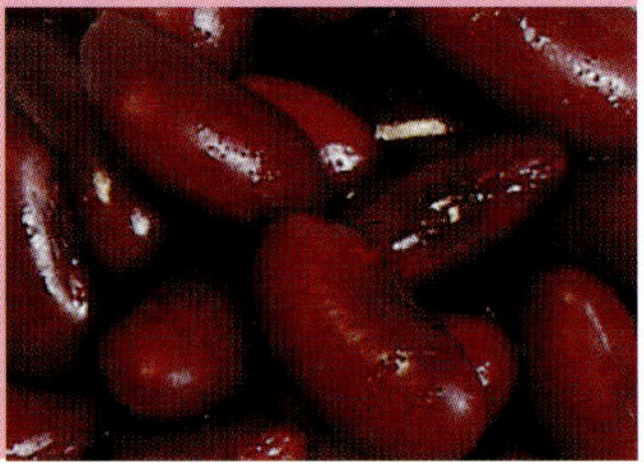

### DIRECTIONS

1. Dry-fry the mince gently in a non-stick frying pan for 3-4 minutes or until well-browned. Remove with a draining spoon.

2. Add the onion to the pan and cook for 4-5 minutes until softened then stir in the garlic and red pepper and cook for a further minute.

3. Return the mince to the pan and add the tomatoes, tomato purée, bay leaf, cumin and chilli. Stir the yeast extract into the stock and add to the pan. Bring to the boil then reduce the heat, cover and cook gently for 20 minutes, stirring occasionally and adding a little further hot stock or water if needed.

4. Add the kidney beans and cook for a further 5-10 minutes.

### RECIPE TIPS

If preferred, you can use pork, chicken or turkey mince for making this recipe. For a vegetarian version, use minced Quorn and a vegetable stock. You can also add extra vegetables such as some chopped mushrooms and / or diced aubergine. Canned chickpeas make an alternative pulse to kidney beans if you happen to have those handy in the cupboard.

## Sardines on Toast

Sardines are an oil-rich fish that provide beneficial omega-3 fatty acids. The canned variety are very convenient to use to make a simple, nutritious light lunch.

SERVES 1

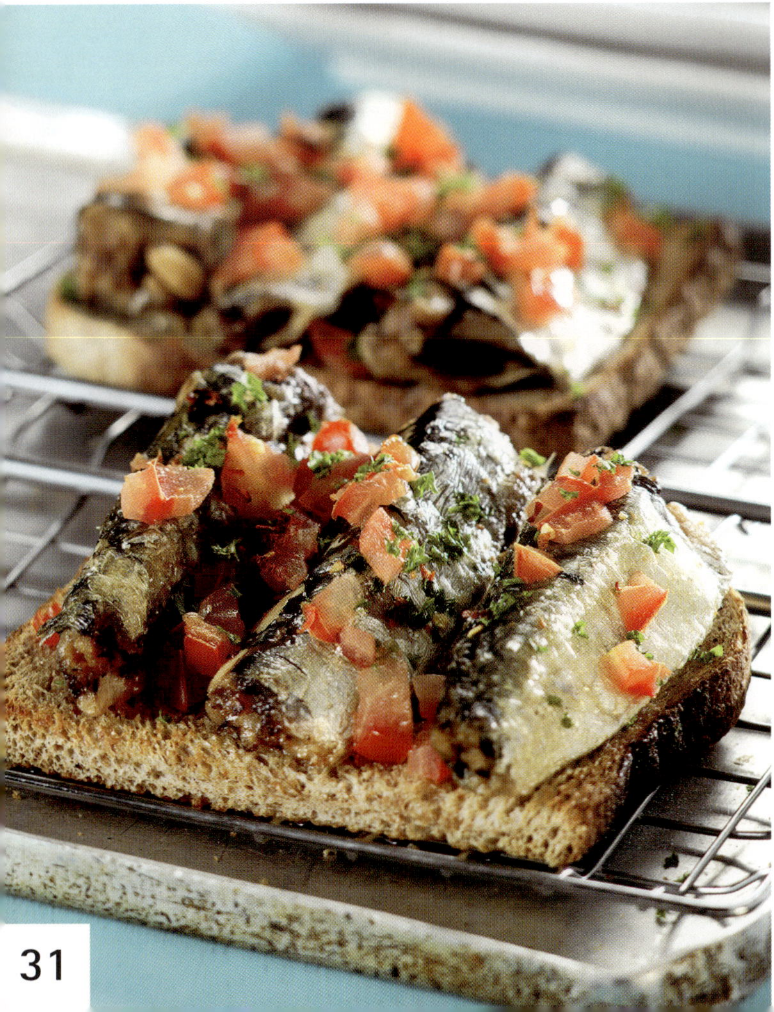

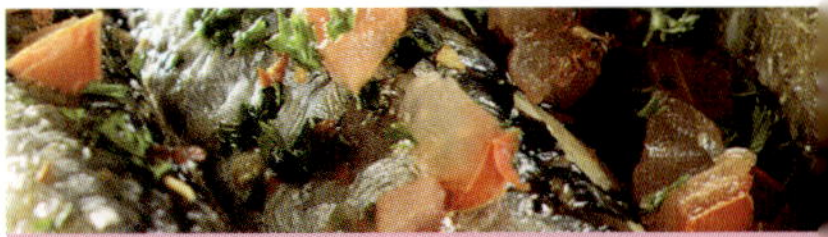

### INGREDIENTS

2 slices wholemeal bread

1 can sardines in olive oil, drained

1 tomato, deseeded and chopped

sprinkling of dried chilli flakes

salt and freshly ground black pepper

1 tbsp chopped fresh parsley, to garnish

### DIRECTIONS

1. Preheat the grill to high. Toast both slices of bread on one side. Turn over and lightly spread the untoasted sides with a little of the drained olive oil from the canned sardines.

2. Arrange the sardines on top of the bread. Top with the chopped tomato and a few chilli flakes. Season to taste. Grill for 3 minutes until golden. Sprinkle with parsley before serving.

## Honey-Glazed Salmon

Salmon is widely available all year round and keenly priced, making it an affordable treat. Here it is marinated in soy, honey and garlic then grilled and sprinkled with toasted sesame seeds. Serve with rice and stir-fried broccoli.

### SERVES 2

### DIRECTIONS

1. Mix together the ingredients for the marinade. Place the salmon in a shallow dish and pour the marinade over. Turn the fish to ensure it is completely covered. Leave to marinate in the refrigerator for at least 1 hour, turning the fish occasionally.

2. Preheat the grill to high. Line the grill pan with foil and place the salmon on top. Brush the fish with the marinade and grill for about 6 minutes, turning once, until just cooked and still pink in the centre.

3. Place the remaining marinade in a small saucepan and heat for 1-2 minutes until thickened and reduced.

4. Spoon the marinade over the salmon before serving and sprinkle with the toasted sesame seeds.

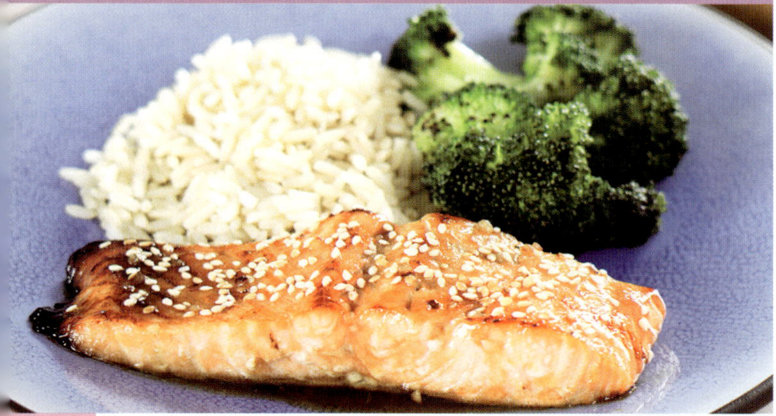

### INGREDIENTS

2 x 150 g (5 oz) salmon fillets, skinned

1 tbsp toasted sesame seeds

### MARINADE

1 garlic clove, crushed

2 tbsp runny honey

1 tbsp soy sauce

1 tbsp sunflower oil

1 tsp toasted sesame oil

### DELICIOUSLY HEALTHY

All fish is good for you but oily fish, such as salmon, mackerel, herring, sardine and trout can actually help to improve your health. These fish are a major source of omega-3 polyunsaturated fatty acids, regular consumption of which can help to reduce the risk of strokes and heart disease and help to improve inflammatory conditions like arthritis. Aim to eat at least one portion of oil-rich fish per week.

## Chicken, Avocado & Rocket Wrap

A tasty and nutritious alternative to a bread sandwich. Lovely for a light lunch.

SERVES 1

### INGREDIENTS

1 small avocado

1 small garlic clove, crushed

squeeze fresh lemon juice

1 tsp reduced-fat mayonnaise

1 tortilla wrap

1 small cooked, chicken breast, skinned and sliced

handful wild rocket leaves

salt and freshly ground black pepper

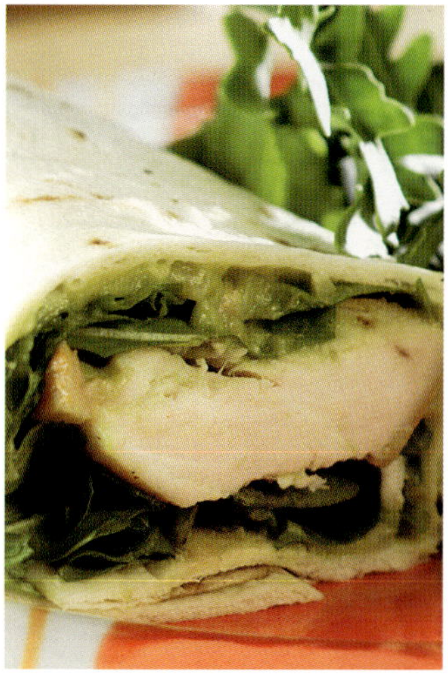

### DIRECTIONS

1. Roughly mash the avocado with the garlic, lemon juice and mayonnaise. Gently warm the tortilla and spread with the avocado mixture.

2. Arrange the chicken and rocket leaves on top. Season, roll up and serve immediately.

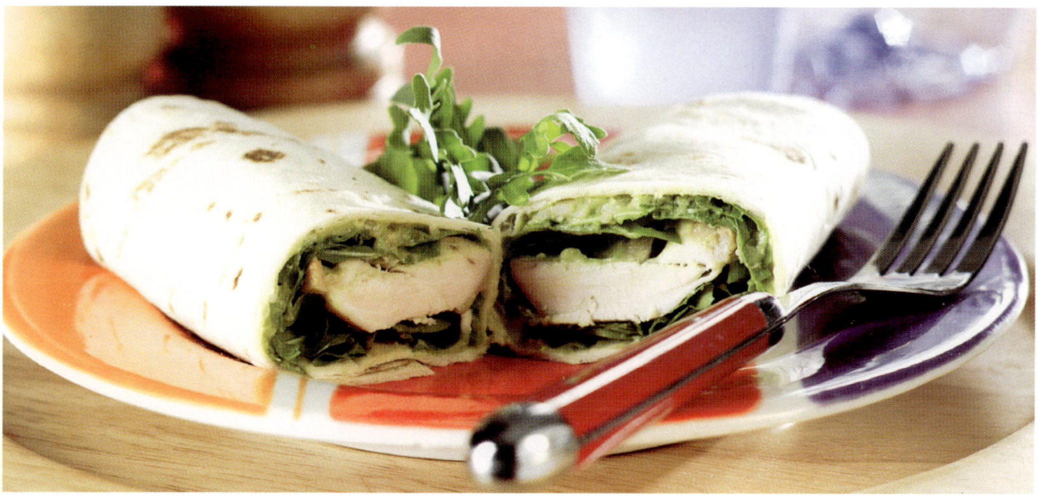

## Ratatouille

A classic medley of Mediterranean flavours packed with vitamins. This makes a delicious vegetable accompaniment or can be tossed with pasta for a quick meal idea.

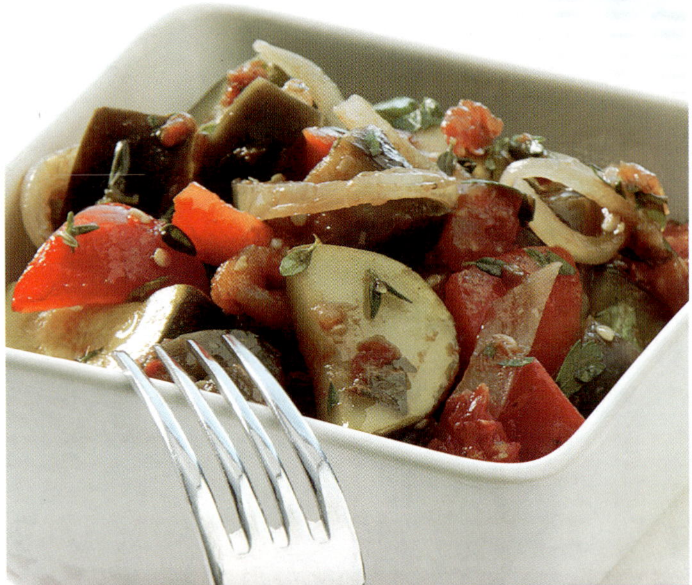

SERVES 4

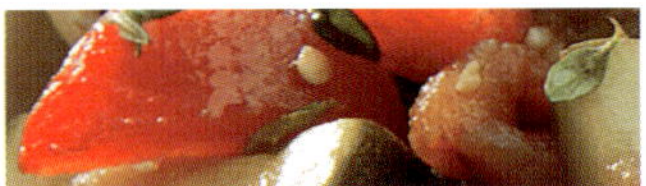

### INGREDIENTS

2 red peppers, deseeded and quartered

2 tbsp vegetable stock

1 onion, very thinly sliced

3 garlic cloves, crushed

2 aubergines, diced

3 courgettes, sliced

400 g (14 oz) canned chopped tomatoes

leaves from a few sprigs each of thyme, marjoram and oregano

freshly ground black pepper

2 tsp olive oil

handful of chopped flat-leaf parsley

handful of shredded basil leaves

### DIRECTIONS

1. Place the peppers under a hot grill and grill, skin-side up, until the skin begins to char. Pop into plastic bag and leave to cool slightly then remove the skin and chop the flesh.

2. Heat the vegetable stock and gently cook the onion and garlic until translucent. Add the aubergines and courgettes, and continue to cook for about 5 minutes. Mix in the red peppers and cook, stirring occasionally, for another minute.

3. Add the tomatoes and snip in the thyme, marjoram and oregano leaves. Season with black pepper.

4. Cover and simmer for about 40 minutes. Stir in the olive oil, parsley and basil and cook, uncovered, for a further 10 minutes until there is no surplus liquid.